# ROGER TROY WILSON'S
# Let's Do Lunch™

WRITE TO SUNSHINE PUBLICATIONS, INC. TO REACH AUTHOR
IN REGARDS TO SPEAKING ENGAGEMENTS OR SEMINARS

First Edition

i

Sunshine Publications, Inc.
23924 Creek Branch Lane
Bonita Springs, FL 34135

Printed and distributed in the United States of America by
The Hanford Press

International Standard Book Number 188488915-8

Library of Congress Catalog Card Number 94-65563

Before I go on, I want to share with you how the name Let's Do Lunch™ came to be. After I had basically finished writing the book, I told my wife I was sure that if I looked in the Bible for the passage where Jesus was feeding the people, the name of the book would come to me. So there I was in bed looking through Matthew, Mark, Luke and John. At the exact Verse where our Precious Savior Jesus was feeding the 5,000 with the little boy's "lunch", the phone rang. It was my mom, saying "Honey, I've got the name of the book - Let's Do Lunch™". I said "Thank you Lord...thank you Jesus...thank you mom!" I think you know exactly how I felt at that moment in time - my cup runneth over!!!

## "I truly believe that Let's Do Lunch™ is a gift from God to all mankind, and without God's gift I would have died from obesity."
Roger Troy Wilson

IN ORDER FOR A DIET TO ACTUALLY WORK FOR THE REST OF YOUR LIFE:

A. You must be able to eat only foods you love, whenever you are hungry and until you are full.

B. You don't have to eat foods you don't like.

C. You have to be able to satisfy your cravings.

D. Unlike other diets, you must not get sick of the foods allowed.

E. You must be able to eat all you want of all the food groups (carbohydrates, fats and proteins) – otherwise your brain will not be satisfied and you will be destined for diet failure.

F. YOU DON'T HAVE TO DO THINGS YOU DON'T LIKE, e.g. exercising, taking pills, counting carbs, calories, points and fat, converting fat grams to calories, measuring or weighing foods, portioning, buying prescribed foods, drinking powdered shakes, attending meetings, etc.

The Let's Do Lunch™ program fulfills all of these necessities.

(The 6'2" author lost 230 pounds and 24 inches from his waist.)

# preface

Allegiance Capital Corporation
12750 Merit Drive, Suite 1410
Dallas, Texas 75251

To: Mr. Roger Troy Wilson

Dear Roger Troy:

Since reading your book, Let's Do Lunch™, I have generated some remarkable results. Several years ago I was diagnosed as a Type 2 Diabetic. Over the years I have tried many different diets without success. Let's Do Lunch™ has not only allowed me to lose 28 pounds, but I have had a remarkable drop in my glucose blood sugar readings. Since being on the Let's Do Lunch™ diet, I have reduced my glucose reading by better than 20%.

In an attempt to control my diabetes, I always shied away from a lot of fruits and drinks like orange juice because of the sugar content. Today my diet is loaded with a variety of sweet fruits, such as grapes, and I have orange juice every morning.

The best part of this diet is I am not hungry nor am I driven by the cravings I have had on previous diets. The combination of learning how to mix fattening and non-fattening foods to lose weight and eating until you are full is certainly unlike other diets I have tried. I have to be honest and state that I have cheated more than once, until I learned how to use some of the substitutes you have recommended. After you are on Let's Do Lunch™ for a few months, your body's metabolism really does change. A few weeks ago I went out for dinner to one of my favorite restaurants and had Veal Marseillaise in a very rich sauce with a side of spaghetti. In the past this had been one of my favorite meals. The intake of rich food didn't sit well with me and I did not feel good for several hours after I ate the meal. It wasn't a pleasant experience. Once you get on the Let's Do Lunch™ diet it is very difficult for you to go back and eat the way you did before.

Your book not only is a boon to dieters everywhere, but as a diabetic, I found it especially beneficial.

Regards,

David J. Mahmood
President and Managing Director
Allegiance Capital Corporation

# dedication

My brother, Steven Neil Wilson, died August 15, 1992, after suffering from terrible stomach cancer. However his death was anything but painful. He sat up in bed, opened his eyes, got the biggest smile on his face I had ever seen, opened his arms as wide as they would go...and at that very moment he died--with the smile still on his face. (He loved Jesus with all of his heart and had been re-baptized in the Pacific Ocean just before his death.)

I want everyone who reads this book to know how very much I loved my brother and how proud I am to have shared his life with him. I believe he will be with me forever as my guardian angel, guiding my endeavors to help save the lives of people all over the world who are losing their battle with obesity, as well as to help those who want to lose a few pounds so that they live healthier and happier lives.

In my brother's name, I am pledging 20 percent of the profits of this book to churches and charities.

Also, I want to thank my wife, Anita, for her support, love, care and concern during all the 400-pound fat years. The same kind of thanks are due my mother and father, Ruth and Orville; my children, Tyra and Ty; my grandchildren, Brandon, Dustin and Brittany; and all the rest of my family, my wife's family and our friends (especially Bob Lichtinger).

My wife tells me she used to worry constantly about me not living and about being alone the rest of her life. And I now know that all my family and friends were embarrassed at times because of my weight, yet none of them ever let on about their unease. For that, I will be forever grateful.

# contents

# CAUTION

CONSULT YOUR PHYSICIAN BEFORE STARTING THE Let's Do Lunch™ EATING PROGRAM.

The publisher and author do not directly or indirectly dispense medical advice or prescribe the use of diet as a form of treatment for sickness without medical approval. Nutritionists and other experts in the field of health and nutrition hold widely varying views. It is not the intent of the publisher or author to diagnose or prescribe. The intent is only to offer information to help you cooperate with your doctor in your mutual quest for health. In the event you use this information without your doctor's approval, you are prescribing for yourself, which is your constitutional right, but the publisher and author assume no responsibility.

Also, because there may be some individual risk involved, the publisher and author are not responsible for any adverse effects or consequences resulting from the use or misuse of any of the requirements, suggestions, preparations, procedures, recipes or other content in this book.

The author is only stating what happened to him, his wife, his mother and his agent, as well as what he believes.

His physicians are Dr. Neil Hoffman of Minneapolis, Minnesota, and Dr. Eli Farri of Fort Myers, Florida. Both witnessed his weight loss.

Please note: Roger Troy Wilson and Sunshine

Further... a comment on exercising: You can lose weight with Let's Do Lunch™ without exercising - or you can lose it even faster by engaging in some physical activity. In any case, the author honestly believes that exercise is beneficial to your health. Try mixing up different activities on different days instead of just one that you do over and over. Just like eating only certain foods that you get sick of after time, the same exercise plan over and over can be boring. Again, please consult your physician to get his/her approval of the activity and/or exercise in which you intend to participate.

Once you have been on Let's Do Lunch™ and get used to the eating changes, you will find that it becomes easier rather than harder. ONCE YOU HAVE READ Let's Do Lunch™, YOU'LL NEVER THINK OF EATING ANY OTHER WAY! There is no better motivation than seeing the weight loss you achieve on your scale.

# chapter one

# From Small to TALL, to Fat, to THIN

As a little kid, my favorite thing to do was to go to Smitty's in La Porte, Indiana, and order a mouth-watering hamburger, deliciously greasy French fries and an extra thick chocolate "frosty malt." Every chance I got, I ended up in a booth at Smitty's with one of my friends, mesmerized in anticipation of the food to come.

Of course, my parents knew about my fixation for this food, and almost every Saturday night after dad's gig (he had a band) they would wake me up by waving one of Smitty's burgers under my nose. I will remember as long as I live how terrific it was to wake up to this scent. (This act of love also endeared me to my mother and father forever.)

Then came my downfall. As a reward for having brought home a good report card, my parents asked if there was anything special I would like. I thought about this for a while and decided I would like them to take me to Smitty's for "all I could eat." They agreed, and I proceeded to take in so many burgers, fries and frosty malts that upon walking outside I upchucked all over the sidewalk. (Of course, this was not what mom and dad expected.) Thus began a tradition; every time I did something good (not miss any school, make the basketball team, get up in the morning), I would ask my parents to take me to Smitty's to "pig out." It was what I wanted, and they consented.

This turned out to be the beginning of my addiction to food.

I ate like a horse and started to become as big as one. But thanks to athletics, I lost what I gained and kept my weight off until I got out of college.

After I married Anita, I stopped working out every day and became the proverbial "couch potato". Unfortunately, my eating habits did not slow down. I gained weight by the week.

The fact that I was depressed because we were very poor didn't help matters. At my lowest moment, I remember Anita trying to cheer me up with the only thing that seemed to give me pleasure (besides her). She surprised me with two family-sized pizzas she had purchased with the last money we had to our names (six very valuable silver dollars that had been handed down to her, generation to generation). I cried, and she hugged me and stroked my hair and told me how much she loved me.

I began to rationalize my food addiction. I only ate when I was happy, sad, satisfied, frustrated, focused, confused, anxious, contented, encouraged, depressed, confident, afraid, loving, etc. I never ran out of reasons for eating.

Within two years I had gained 100 pounds.

I ate almost nonstop, from the time I got home from work until I went to bed. And I ate everything you can imagine: hamburgers, hot dogs, tacos, nachos with cheese, french fries, milk shakes, sub sandwiches, fried chicken, fried fish, cheesecake, ice cream, chocolate bars, cashews, etc.

I also ate throughout my workdays. I remember innumerable business luncheons when I actually told the waitress to serve me two full meals, one right after the other. (I don't have to tell you how often my expense account was questioned.)

Over the years, I paid a painful price for my compulsive behavior.

I remember going to the "big and tall" clothing store and praying they had something in my size. I had a 5-foot waist and a 22-inch neck, and many times the shop simply didn't have anything in inventory to fit me. I felt like a freak.

When I was in first class on an airplane and the stewardess had to bring me a seat belt extension, I was so embarrassed that I put my face in a magazine for the whole trip.

Then there were all the times we went out to eat and everyone wanted to sit in a booth, but I just wouldn't fit. I could see the looks on the faces of the people around us as they snickered and whispered about my weight. I can't begin to tell you how bad I hurt when this happened. But I just couldn't help myself – I still sat down at a table and stuffed my big fat face.

It seems like yesterday when I drove a golf cart and ended up with everyone in the clubhouse staring at the long black mark on my shirt, caused by the steering wheel rubbing against my enormous belly. After I noticed the eyeing, I sat there the whole time with my arms crossed over the mark. I snuck out through the back door and went home feeling totally lost as to what to do about my problem.

I also remember my embarrassment at an amusement park, when everyone watched as I could not lock myself into the roller coaster and had to get up and leave. I went off by myself, unable to hold back the tears.

Then, there was the day I had to sit on one side of our friends' boat while everyone else sat on the other side. I didn't say a word as I anxiously awaited the end of the ride, and I never accepted an invitation like that again.

At a University of Minnesota wine-tasting party for the benefit of the Williams Scholarship Fund, I won the drawing for "your weight in wine." The master of ceremonies said, "Oh my ____, I don't believe it. The winner weighs 360 pounds." My face turned beet red as I walked to the podium. I wanted to crawl under a table.

Even when I never expected it, my weight became a humiliation. My doctor (Neil Hoffman of Minneapolis, Minnesota) had put me in the hospital for three days to give me a thorough physical. The very first evening, while I was lying on my bed, I heard a loud, squeaky noise coming down the hall. Closer and closer it came to my room. Finally the door swung open as two nurses (soaked in perspiration) wheeled in the hospital freight scale and asked me to please get on. I felt like a steer going to market. At that moment, I actually hated myself.

Although my eating was out of control, I desperately tried again and again to get a handle on it.

I attempted so many diets that it *almost* became funny to me, so much so that I went around telling my friends I was going to write a book called "How To Gain And Maintain, by R. T. Wilson, President of the

Tons of Fun Weight Club." It was going to say things like, "You must have chocolate during sex, in order to make up for the calories being burned," and "Hamburgers are a must at the end of a gourmet evening, because you'll still be starving." This humor was really a mask for my heavy-heartedness.

I was a professional "diet failure". I just didn't have the discipline and willpower necessary to succeed. Following are a few examples of my futile attempts:

- For about two weeks, I followed a diet that involved measuring and weighing food, food exchanges, and a weekly weighing in and meeting. The problem was I just didn't feel like I got enough to eat. (Even though this program undoubtedly works for a lot of people, it just didn't work for me.)

- I was on a high protein and fat diet, eating cheese, bacon, eggs, meat, butter, etc., and lost some weight over a few weeks. But even though it worked, I got sick of eating all the greasy food that was prescribed and not being able to eat other foods. So, I gradually started eating in my old way and ended up fat again.

- Then I tried a liquid diet. I drank powders mixed in water and learned about nutrition. Once again, even though this program undoubtedly works for a lot of people, it just didn't work for me. I lasted about three weeks, until at a University of Minnesota basketball game I told my wife I felt very weird, like I was in a twilight zone. She said, "Forget it. This diet might be causing more harm than it's worth." I was off and eating again.

- It got to where I was desperate and would try just about anything. For instance, our daughter's mother-in-law and I went to an acupuncture specialist who stuck needles in our heads. This was supposed to cure her smoking problem and, of course, my weight problem. On our way home from the treatment, we looked at each other and started laughing. She lit up a cigarette and drove me to the doughnut shop.

- Another time I decided it was only necessary to *taste* the foods I liked. So, without anyone knowing about it, I went to McDonald's® and bought three Quarter Pounder® burgers with cheese, two large orders of fries, two chocolate shakes, a cherry pie and an apple pie. I then went into my bedroom and proceeded to chew the food and not swallow anything. That's right, I used an airline bag every time I tasted something. This shows just how badly I wanted to lose weight (unfortunately, it also shows my intelligence level).

- Along came our daughter Tyra's wedding and nothing ever motivated me more to lose weight. And nothing I ever did before, or have done since, was more painful than losing the weight I lost in order to proudly walk her down the aisle. I literally, agonizingly pushed myself away from the table for 9 months and got down to 278 pounds. I was so proud of myself! But, the day of the wedding, even as I was walking her down the aisle, all I could think about was pigging out at the reception.

Can you imagine not being able to enjoy your own daughter's wedding, because your mind had been tortured for so long that it was monopolized by its desire for foods it had been deprived of? That night my brain became satisfied as I ate and drank everything in sight. I was off and eating again and gained all the weight back, plus more.

Then (play it again, Sam) I got sick of the way I looked, and almost every Monday I'd start dieting again – trying to duplicate what I did for Tyra's wedding, yet tormenting my brain.

This would last sometimes a day and sometimes two or three, and then I would offer Anita or our son, Ty, money to go get a family-size pizza, lots of tacos and nachos with cheese, cashews, chocolate covered peanuts, chips and dip, cake, ice cream, chocolate bars – you name it and I bribed a member of my family to go get it for me. Then, after gorging myself until I couldn't eat anymore, I would say to my wife, "Throw all the rest of this stuff away because I'm starting my diet tomorrow." Starting a diet the next day, of course, never happened. Anita got smart and wouldn't throw the food away. Instead, she would hide it from me so that when I asked for it again she would already have it and wouldn't have to spend money just to appease my appetite.

She tells me today that the reason she always went to the store to get what I wanted was simply that, even though it hurt her terribly, she couldn't stand for me to be unhappy.

In my later fat years, because of all my embarrassments and humiliations, I became a "closet eater". When eating out, I would eat just like everyone else, and when I got home I would satiate myself with everything fattening I could get my hands on.

Then, with the help of our Father in Heaven, I ended up developing a diet that actually allows me to eat until I'm full, foods we all love, whenever I'm hungry and without doing anything distasteful – no exercising, no pills, no shakes, no counting carbs, calories, fats or points, no converting fat grams to calories, no measuring or weighing food, no portioning, no prescribed foods to buy, no chemicals to take, no specific liquids to drink and no meetings to attend.

In fact, I actually lost my weight by eating foods we all love until I was completely full and could not eat any more...and, to the best of my knowledge, I became the only formerly obese person in the world to have written a diet book and kept the weight off!

After I started losing weight, my wife couldn't believe it because I ate so much food and didn't exercise. She actually thought there was something wrong with me. She thought I was sick - and I don't mean mentally.

She didn't say anything about her concern right away, however, because she was so happy to see the weight come off.

Several things happened while I was losing weight. My blood pressure went down "on the low side" from 90+ to between 60 and 80. I got rid of my apnea and snoring. My hips and feet stopped hurting. My acid indigestion left me. My face became thinner without any major sagging of the skin. My potassium level rose naturally. My skin stayed soft and smooth. And *my stomach shrank, even though I was eating until I was completely full and couldn't eat any more.* Because my stomach had shrunk, I couldn't eat as much as I did before. (I developed what I believe is the only way to speed up the body's metabolism naturally – no exercising, no pills and no chemicals.)

I also found that it didn't matter where I ate my food. I continued to lie on my bed, on my side, and eat.

Anita, however, continued to worry that I was sick. After I had lost approximately 190 pounds, again *without exercising,* she actually thought that cancer was the reason for my weight loss and made me have a physical. Our dear friend, Dr. Eli Farri of Fort Myers, Florida, said I was fine and sent me home to tell her that whatever I was doing, I should continue doing it.

She cried.

Shortly after that, she said, "Honey, please don't

lose any more weight; you look just perfect." *I don't have to tell you how proud I was!*

Up until this time, my thinking was that alcohol would curtail my weight loss; therefore, I had abstained.  Now, with Anita's pronouncement that I was perfect and shouldn't lose any more weight, I decided to start drinking socially again.  The idea that I should drink "only wines" came to me in the middle of the night.  (It wasn't the first time I'd had such an "awakening."  In fact, almost the whole Let's Do Lunch™ diet was a result of God's awakenings.)  So, I started drinking wines, in addition to all the food I was eating.  I lost another 40 pounds.  (In retrospect, although weight loss is more dramatic when alcohol is eliminated, I maintain it is not necessary to abstain in order to lose weight.  You just lose more slowly if you decide to have some wine now and then.)

Anita was astounded and insisted I have *another* physical.  Dr. Farri had to call and assure her there was nothing wrong with me.  *I don't have to tell you how pleased she was.*  She looked at me like I was the most wonderful china doll she had ever seen.

And here's the coup de grace. Anita actually asked me if I thought she could lose 8 pounds on Let's Do Lunch™ (the 8 pounds she had not been able to lose all of her adult life).  She didn't believe she could eat so much food and still lose weight.  To make a long story short, she didn't lose the 8 pounds – she lost 23 pounds and is thinner now than she was at age 18.

My mother, after watching me eat to my heart's content, said, "Honey, have you gone off your diet?" I told her that the way I was eating was the way I always eat on my diet, and I then asked if she was interested in losing any weight. She started Let's Do Lunch™, lost 51 pounds and went from a size 18 to a size 10, *without exercise of any kind!*

I've told you about some of the terribly embarrassing experiences I had when I was heavy. Now I'd like to tell you about some of the marvelous experiences I've had as a thin man.

The foremost occasions that come to mind (and are a little embarrassing and yet very gratifying for me to relate) are the numerous times people actually thought I was a movie star or a TV personality. The first time it happened was in a restaurant in Louisville, Kentucky. Anita and I noticed everyone staring at us. Then the manager walked up, excused himself for interrupting and said he knew who I was but was sorry he couldn't remember my name. I told him I was sorry, but I couldn't recall ever having met him. He said we'd never met, but he'd seen me in the movies and on television. I told him I was flattered, but I wasn't who he thought I was. He said he understood my not wanting to be bothered, but he just wanted to thank us for dining with them. He told us we'd made their day, and he hoped we would enjoy ourselves enough to come back and see them again. I didn't know what to say, so I just thanked him for the kind words and told him if we ever came back to Louisville we would definitely stop and say hello. I was really embarrassed, but also gloating inside – and Anita never heard the end of it.

Then there was the episode at the jam-packed movie studio amusement park, when the casting director for their mock TV show selected our son, Ty, to be the announcer. I remember Ty looking at me and winking, like, "Ha, ha, Dad, I got the part." Then, right after he went through the dressing room door, the casting director selected me to be the "leading man, main guest."

As I entered the dressing room Ty looked up at me in astonishment and said, "What are you doing here?" When I told him, he just shook his head in disbelief - and HE has never heard the end of it.

I remember calling three of my old working buddies and arranging a luncheon. I drove to downtown St. Paul and as I was parking my car I saw one of them doing the same. I didn't say a thing as we walked side by side into the restaurant. He had looked right at me *and had no idea who I was!* I turned toward him and asked if he had a match (I have no idea why I asked for a match, since I don't smoke). He replied that he did not. I then said, "Well, you really ought to have a match for one of your old best buddies." He looked at me again and stared. At last, he recognized me. His mouth dropped open and he was absolutely speechless. Finally, he threw his arms around me and said, "My _____, I don't believe it!" It was all I could do to hold back the tears.

Even my best friend from high school didn't

recognize me. When I arranged to meet him at a California hotel, my wife, my parents and I got there early and sat where we could see everyone coming in, yet they could not see us. As my pal arrived, I got up and walked toward him. We looked at each other and he continued walking right past me. I turned around and followed him, as he was obviously looking for me. When he didn't see the "old" me, he proceeded to a pay phone to make a call. I stood a few feet away and stared. He dropped his eyes to avoid my stare and placed his call. He looked up, saw that I was still staring at him and said, "Is there something I can help you with, sir?" I said, "Well, you could help me find my best high school buddy." After what I said registered, his expression changed to shock and he dropped the phone. He was speechless as he threw his arms around me. We joined my wife and my parents and talked and talked and talked. Several times during the conversation he stopped just to stare at me. I felt like I had won the lottery.

Blood relatives, too, didn't know who I was. In a bar at the Cleveland airport between planes, I heard a voice I recognized. I said, "Shelly?" She looked at me, and when she didn't recognize me she said in a quizzical manner, "Yes?" I just stared at her, and she looked at me and said, "Do I know you?" I said, "Well, you should – I've been your cousin since you were born." She stared at me for the longest time and finally said, "Roger Troy?" I said, "Yes," and she threw her arms around me and SCREAMED, "Oh my _____!" Several times during the conversation that followed, she looked at me and lost her train of thought. I had to pry myself away in order to catch my plane.  When I reached the gate, I turned around and there she was. She had followed me and just stood there in a daze. Later, I found out she called family members around the country to tell them I looked like a movie star (boy, were my buttons ever popping when I heard about this).

And, just imagine how it felt for me to attend my high school class reunion sporting a svelte body – especially since I had gotten progressively heavier at each of the previous ones.  I had planned to not walk in with my wife.  People were looking at me and wondering who I was.  Finally, one classmate came over and asked if I was the guest speaker.  Absolutely no one had even an inkling as to my identity.  What a commotion I caused!  And what an absolutely marvelous time I had showing off my thinness and dancing with my old girlfriends.  I was the talk of the town.  It was my proudest moment.

By now you have probably wondered if any problems resulted from my incredible weight loss. There was only one:  I had an apron of skin hanging from my tummy.  Even though I could have lived with this the rest of my life, it bothered me.  So, I chose to have a tummy tuck.  I interviewed several plastic surgeons and selected Dr. William Carter of Edina Plastic Surgery (Edina, Minnesota) to make the necessary cuts (approximately 50 percent of the way around my body).  Because of my previous massive size, Dr. Carter also tightened all the muscles in my stomach. Upon viewing his masterpiece, he looked at his nurse and said, "Look at that - he looks like a 25-year old". I *have absolutely never, ever been so happy about anything in my life!* To have a board for a tummy, after living with a 5-foot waist, is the most triumphant feeling you can imagine.

Of course, prior to my tummy tuck I needed a medical examination in order to insure that I was physically able to have surgery. This "pre-op" exam was done by my friend, Dr. Neil Hoffman of Minneapolis, Minnesota.

A few days after surgery, I received the following letter from him:

Dear Roger:

I hope the surgery went well. I just wanted to let you know that your blood count was normal, your urinalysis looked good, and your cholesterol is 158. TELL ANITA THE BAD NEWS IS THIS MEANS YOU'RE GOING TO LIVE A LONG TIME. All your blood fats look good. Your blood sugar, liver, kidney and bone function studies are normal. So just a quick note to let you know that all of your laboratory studies including your coagulation studies, thyroid, blood fats all look normal and that I hope things went well. I look forward to seeing you again.

Most sincerely,

NEIL R. HOFFMAN, M.D., F.A.C.P.

## chapter two

# The Grapes Of Weight

I'll always remember that fateful day when by accident my life was changed forever. I remember it like it was yesterday. It was a beautiful October day and I was in my summer home in Minneapolis, Minnesota, watching TV. I decided (as was usual for a 425 pound guy) it was "pig-out time". So, for the 15,000th time in my life I went to the kitchen to find something to eat – maybe cookies and coffee, or cake and ice cream, or a big chocolate bar.

I opened the freezer and, to my surprise, found some grapes. They were ruined – frozen solid. I accused Anita, and she said she didn't do it.

Aha! The culprit had to be our son, Ty. I blame him for everything, even if he's not in town.

I called him at Billiard Street Cafe™ in Fridley, Minnesota (he and his partner own the place) and told him, "Hey, son, when you're over at our house, please have the common courtesy to not ruin our food."

Ty then told me the grapes were not ruined; that I obviously had never eaten frozen grapes; that they were a great snack food and had the texture of a Popsicle®; that the freezing enhanced the sweetness; and that they were surely much better for me than all the garbage I normally ate.

I put a frozen grape in my mouth, bit into it and loved it. It was cold, made my mouth feel good, and somehow the freezing did enhance the sweetness. (Thank you, son.)

After eating frozen grapes until they were coming out my ears, I decided I didn't want any more. It is important that you realize what I'm saying here. I literally ate so many grapes that I was sick of them and just couldn't eat any more. I'm talking pounds of them. Thousands of calories of them. So I went to the kitchen to get something else to eat – maybe some chips and dip, or maybe a family-size pizza or something. But lo and behold, I didn't WANT anything else. This had never happened before. I wasn't hungry, so I went to bed.

The next evening the same thing happened - EXACTLY! That's when I decided to eat frozen grapes every night (instead of junk food) while watching TV. After about a month, my clothes were loose. I obviously had lost a few pounds even though I was eating thousands of calories of frozen grapes each night, and even though I was still drinking and eating in my same old fattening way at dinner time.

NOTE: Let's Do Lunch™ IS NOT A FRUIT DIET!

It involves sometimes eating a little fruit, but that's only the beginning! And don't worry if you can't tolerate, or simply don't like, certain fruits. This part of the program works because *you choose the fruits you eat*, and you can eat canned fruits. (If you have physical problems, like colitis or diabetes, see your doctor for a list of fruits that are acceptable.)

Further, let me shock you right off the bat – no matter what anyone says, after 15 years of experimenting with my own body IT IS MY BELIEF THAT FRUIT SUGAR (FRUCTOSE) IS NON-FATTENING – NO MATTER HOW MANY CALORIES ARE INVOLVED, whereas refined and processed sugars are extremely fattening – even though they have no fat grams in them – and diet sweeteners cause cravings for all the wrong foods.

Also, to keep you interested, Let's Do Lunch™ INCLUDES burgers, steaks, baked beans, corn on the cob, barbecue chicken, glazed salmon, Caesar salads, omelets, grapes, sloppy joes, stuffed peppers, chicken Parmesan, chili, tuna salad, meatloaf and many other foods you probably would never think of eating until full while trying to lose weight.

Read on, and be sure to consult your physician before starting the Let's Do Lunch™ eating program.

Needless to say, soon after I figured out I could eat pounds of frozen grapes every evening and lose weight, I started to wonder whether I could eat oodles of other fruits and lose weight. So, I started eating as much as I wanted of all different kinds of fruits (in place of my normal evening junk food). I ate mangos, kiwi, watermelon, cantaloupe, melon, strawberries, pears, apples, plums, honeydew, oranges, tangerines, peaches and, of course, grapes until they were coming out of my ears. To give you an idea of the volume of fruit I ate, at one sitting I consumed half a watermelon, a whole cantaloupe, four tangerines, four plums, two apples and then finished it off with a pound of grapes. And I lost weight.

I was on a roll. I was losing weight and it was easy. Now I wanted to lose it even faster. I started thinking about eliminating all the fattening drinks and foods I was eating at mealtimes. You know, just eat veggies, soups, salads, lean meat, chicken, turkey and fish from now on. Of course, I had tried that many times before – unsuccessfully. (Most of these foods taste awful when prepared in a dietary way.)

Soon after that, in the middle of the night, God

woke me up with an idea:  if I didn't like something that was non-fattening, why not add a little something fattening to make it taste great.  It was worth a try.

Here are some of the strategies I came up with:

- Grill, broil, bake, or blacken the fish, and dip my fork in on-the-side tartar sauce (made with Hellmann's® Reduced Fat cholesterol free mayonnaise dressing and sweet relish).  Delicious - and I ate all the fish I wanted and still lost weight.  Again, it's important that you understand what I just said:  I didn't eat just 3-1/2 ounces of grilled or blackened fish; I ate three or four whole fillets.

- Fry extra lean hamburger and ground turkey breast together – mix with pinto beans, add chopped onions and heat (about 1/2 pinto beans, 1/4 hamburger and 1/4 ground turkey breast).  I loved it (the turkey takes on the taste of the hamburger).  I ate to my heart's content, dipping my fork in on-the-side ketchup, mustard, relish, onions, etc.  And I lost weight.

- Prepare a salad with three-bean salad on top, peas, corn, onion, tomato, beets and green pepper, adding a small portion of my all-time favorite (blue cheese) and dip my fork in on-the-side reduced-calorie French dressing or a Newman's Own® dressing.  Once more, it was delicious, *and I ate all I wanted and still lost weight.*

- Melt (in the microwave) two slices of Borden™ fat-free sharp nonfat process cheese product on a large package of mixed veggies. I loved it, and I ate all I wanted and still lost weight.

- Bring home hot barbecue chicken from the grocery store, take the skin off and eat the meat with three-bean salad (also bought at the store and with as much of the oil as possible drained off). I'd eat the whole chicken and a quart of three-bean salad, while my wife watched in astonishment! And I lost weight.

- Make my omelet without cheese, but with tomato, green pepper and onion, and eat it with salsa. Sometimes I'd savor a six-egg monstrosity!

- Make my chili with half extra lean ground beef and half ground turkey breast (fried together, using 100% extra virgin olive oil cooking spray). Outstanding, and I lost weight. Three or four large bowls full normally did the trick. (The turkey took on the flavor of the ground beef.)

- Drink my coffee with skim milk, instead of the cream I normally used.

YOU GET THE IDEA.

I was now drinking mostly diet iced tea and eating veggies, soups, salads, red meat, chicken, turkey and fish at meal times; and I drank and ate all I wanted (not just 3-1/2 oz. of fish, etc.). I was losing weight, my way.

For those meals when I wanted just a little something to eat, here are a couple of my favorites:

- Store-bought sliced baked turkey, with a slice of Kraft® fat-free cheese melted on it and served on a slice of Wasa® light rye original crispbread (this bread looks like a huge cracker and is fat-free). I ate anywhere from one to four of these.

- Tuna salad, made with just enough Hellmann's® Reduced Fat cholesterol free mayonnaise dressing to hold it together. Put this on a slice of Wasa® light rye original crispbread, along with tomato, sweet relish and onion. Again, I ate one to four.

And here's what will blow your mind: my stomach shrank, even though I was eating tremendous volumes of food.

Today, as I'm typing this, there is absolutely no way I could eat the volumes of food I ate when I first started Let's Do Lunch™. How could I? After all, my stomach shrank 24 inches.

Keep in mind that many distinguished people, including my family doctors, witnessed my weight loss.

Remember, too, that Let's Do Lunch™ caused my own mother to lose all her weight. She went from a size 18 dress to a size 10 – WITHOUT EXERCISE OF ANY KIND.

And for those of you who have only a few pounds to

lose, let me remind you about my own wife's loss of 23 pounds when she only wanted to lose the 8 pounds she had not been able to lose all of her adult life. She is 5 feet 7 inches tall and had never been overweight. But she wanted to lose those eight pounds. She was hesitant about even trying my program – simply because she didn't believe she could eat that much food and take in that many calories and still lose weight.

She asked, "Honey, do you think I could go on Let's Do Lunch™ and lose the eight pounds I've always wanted to lose?" "What's the worst that can happen?" I asked her. "If it doesn't work for you, simply go back to what you have been doing. No harm, no foul." She decided to Let's Do Lunch™ and she didn't lose the 8 pounds – SHE LOST 23 POUNDS!

Lest you think that what I have told you so far is all there is to it – NOT. You'll have to read on, especially to memorize God's key that makes it all work – and I believe speeds up the body's metabolism naturally – no exercising, no pills and no chemicals. You'll also find out about nonfat foods that I believe are fattening, fattening foods that I believe are non-fattening, how to deal with cravings, eating out, grocery shopping, fixing meals, buying food "to go" and what I did in place of exercising.

Now let's discuss our society's eating habits!

How dumb can we get – eating our big meal of the day just before going to bed, so all that food just lays there, all night long, in a dormant body, and most of it turns to fat!  Think about it – the body should be active after eating the big meal of the day, in order to burn all the food we have eaten.

How much dumber can we get – getting up in the morning and trying to eat lightly all day long, so we can pig-out at night and get fatter!

The dumbest – after not eating all night long, trying to eat lightly all day long subjects us to terrible cravings for snacks, and when we snack it almost always is on something fattening!  And, after eating something fattening, we all feel like we have "blown it" so, why watch what we eat – at least for the rest of that day.

Thinking about it logically, when should your big meal of the day occur?  As I've already explained, not at night – and not at breakfast, because breakfast food will digest long before the day is through and you will end up eating another big meal at dinnertime.

Therefore,

### "LET'S DO LUNCH"™
(God's key to opening your diet door
for the rest of your life)

NOTE: Remember to consult your physician before
starting.

You will want to memorize the rest of this chapter and follow it for two weeks, after which time it will have become a habit.

It's quite simple. To start with, the amount of food you eat each day should not be cut down. You will just be eating in a smarter way.

## BREAKFAST

Try to eat only a little fresh fruit, like an apple, 1/2 grapefruit or a fruit smoothie (read on for recipe) for breakfast TO SPEED UP YOUR METABOLISM. It is my belief that fruits digest faster than any other foods and therefore, if eaten by themselves, speed up the body's metabolism naturally. If fresh fruit is not available, then canned (in fruit juices) is okay.

NOTE: If you crave cereal for breakfast, read on to find out how you can eliminate this craving.

Then, if possible, eat nothing throughout the rest of the morning, SO THAT BY LUNCHTIME YOU ARE FAMISHED!

REMEMBER:

- Only a little fresh fruit or a fruit smoothie at breakfast speeds up your metabolism.

- Eat nothing the rest of the morning so you will have a big appetite at lunch.

## "LET'S DO LUNCH"™

Then, Let's Do Lunch™ – Your big meal of the day!

**(Don't worry if you can't eat your big meal of the day at lunchtime ...just read on.)**

Let's Do Lunch™ is "ALL YOU CAN EAT" of as lean as possible red meat, chicken, turkey, fish and other acceptable proteins, along with "all you can eat" of acceptable soups, salads, vegetables, etc. The following chapters will explain how to add something fattening to each of these foods – when eating out and at home – in order for you to thoroughly enjoy each and every Let's Do Lunch™.

For example, you will be able to eat lean steaks, lean hamburger, baked beans, corn on the cob, popcorn, barbecue chicken, grapes, glazed salmon, Caesar salads, omelets, tuna salad, chili, chicken Parmesan, beef stew, taco salad, barbecue beef, egg salad, bean soup, chicken salad, coleslaw, chicken chow mein, three-bean salad, stuffed peppers, meatloaf (all healthy foods), and many other foods you probably would never think of eating until full while trying to lose weight...and you can eat them with all the regular sauces and condiments, e.g. ketchup, mustard, tartar sauce, etc!

It is imperative that you eat a generous portion of protein (protein keeps you satisfied longer) for each and every Let's Do Lunch™, so you won't get terrible cravings for snacks in the afternoon and for all the wrong foods at dinnertime!

NOTE:  If you have cravings for breads, pasta, potatoes and cereals, be sure to eat some special salsa, antipasto, corn on the cob, popcorn, or something with corn, beans or peas in it – in order to ELIMINATE these cravings. (You must satisfy your cravings and this will be explained in the next chapter.)

After Let's Do Lunch™, if possible, eat nothing more until dinnertime.

REMEMBER:

- Let's Do Lunch™ is "ALL YOU CAN EAT" and includes a generous portion of protein ... so you won't go off your diet later in the day.

- Because you have had all you can eat, you will NOT need to snack in the afternoon.

# **DINNER**

For dinner, eat as much as you can of only fruits. Fresh fruit is much better for you, but if fresh is not available then canned – in fruit juice – is okay, again speeding up your metabolism. Sometimes I eat just grapes or frozen grapes until I am totally satisfied, or I fix a fruit smoothie by blending 1/2 dozen ice cubes and 1-1/2 cups of unsweetened orange, pineapple or apple juice with 1/2 of a frozen banana and other fresh fruit. If I substitute unsweetened frozen fruit, I add water for the correct consistency, instead of ice cubes. These drinks are very soothing and satisfying.

NOTE:  Peel and cut bananas in half and freeze in
             freezer bags, for use in smoothies.

If, after eating only fruits or fruit smoothies for dinner you are still not satisfied, then eat acceptable soups, salads, vegetables, special salsa, antipasto, corn on the cob, popcorn, or something with beans, peas or corn in it until you are satisfied – BUT NO PROTEINS. Remember, your big meal of the day is Let's Do Lunch™.

REMEMBER:

- At dinner eat as much fruit as you can – preferably fresh, canned in fruit juices is okay, or drink fruit smoothies.

- If after the fruit you are still not satisfied, wait 1/2 hour and eat the other foods listed above –

BUT NO PROTEINS.

Think about it – which is better, laying dormant in bed all night with only fast-digesting non-fattening foods to metabolize, or laying there with your stomach chock-full of slow-digesting fattening foods that I believe will mostly turn into body-fat when the body is not active?

- If you get the "munchies" during the middle of the night, eat some fresh fruit, fruit salad or a fruit smoothie. (Anita and I have a small box of Sun-Maid® Raisins on each of the end tables in our bedroom, so we can satisfy our "sweet tooth" at any time.)

## "LET'S DO LUNCH"™ AT DINNERTIME

If you are a person who cannot do Let's Do Lunch™ at lunchtime, then Let's Do Lunch™ should be eaten at dinnertime, eating all the fruit you can for lunch – followed by acceptable soups, salads, vegetables, special salsa, antipasto, corn on the cob, popcorn, or something with beans, peas or corn in it...BUT NO PROTEINS FOR LUNCH! If fruit is not available for lunch, or if you just don't feel like eating any fruit for lunch, it's OKAY...just eat the other foods and skip the fruit.

Then **just prior to eating your Let's Do Lunch**™

(including your only protein of the day) at dinnertime, eat all the fruit you can (again...unless you just don't feel like eating any fruit).

If you miss lunch entirely, just follow the paragraph immediately above.

REMEMBER:

- When Let's Do Lunch™ is going to be eaten at dinnertime, at lunch eat only fruit and/or other acceptable foods -  BUT NO PROTEINS.

- Just before eating Let's Do Lunch™ (including your only protein of the day) at dinnertime, eat all the fresh fruit you can.

- At a dinner party, eat the nonfattening foods and the proteins and say "no thank you" to dessert.

## NOTES:

1. If "only fruit for breakfast" just doesn't do it for you, immediately upon waking eat just a little fruit to get your "metabolism motor" started.  Then, after getting ready for work, eat as small a breakfast as possible, e.g. an egg or two, or (for those cereal eaters who need a car-

bohydrate fix) a soy protein shake – blending a half-dozen ice cubes and 1-1/2 cups of unsweetened orange, pineapple or apple juice with 1/2 package of KetoSlim® protein powder, 1/2 of a frozen banana and other fresh fruit. If you substitute unsweetened frozen fruit, add water for the correct consistency, instead of ice cubes. (Peel and cut bananas in half and freeze in freezer bags, for use in smoothies.)

2. On those days when you are famished in the morning, go ahead and have as much fresh fruit for breakfast as you want. (Dr. Michael Criqui and others at the University of California, San Diego, Medical Center found that people who lived longest ate the most fresh fruit.)

NOTE: **It is imperative that you eat some fruit each and every day – if you don't, you will get terrible cravings for foods with processed sugar (regular sugar) in them and end up going off your diet.**

**Always remember that it is my belief that <u>PROCESSED SUGAR IS 100% FATTENING</u> (even though there are no fat grams in it), whereas fructose (sugar from fruits) is 100% non-fattening.** Therefore, go to the health food store and buy fructose to use in your cooking, drinks, etc.

3. **When eating Let's Do Lunch™ out, order**

protein, soup, salad, vegetables, etc. and order an extra portion of just the protein, so you won't get terrible cravings for snacks in the afternoon and for all the wrong foods at dinnertime. For example, eat your "blackened chicken Caesar salad" with an extra portion of "blackened chicken" and, of course, without croutons.

4. Force yourself to eat a big Let's Do Lunch™, including the generous portion of protein (protein keeps you satisfied longer), so you won't go off your diet.

5. Don't eat fruit between "daytime meals"..if you do, you will eventually get sick of eating fruits and go off your diet.

Also, if you eat fruit immediately following any meal it could cause an "upset stomach" - try to wait 2 hours.

If you get the "munchies" from 2 hours after dinner until breakfast the next morning, eat some fresh fruit, fruit salad or a fruit smoothie.

6. The longer you can wait to have lunch, the less you will be able to eat for dinner, and therefore the weight will come off even faster.

7. If you change nothing else, make sure your only protein of the day is eaten with your Let's Do Lunch™ meal. You should lose weight and

live a healthier and happier life!

8. The one thing that can definitely knock you off your diet is drinking. It won't happen every time you drink ... but every time you drink the odds go up that it will happen. Try to abstain, but if you just can't, and the inevitable does happen, remember to do my "fruit and soup flush" the next day. (I'll explain later.)

****** NOW GO BACK AND READ FROM **"BREAK-FAST"** ON, AGAIN AND AGAIN ... UNTIL YOU HAVE IT MEMORIZED!

## chapter three

# Cravings, Eating Out and Other Diet Dilemmas

Note:    To start with, throw away all the fattening foods you have in your home (see the Grocery Shopping chapter for acceptable foods).  This is an investment in your weight loss and your family's health. Your entire family will love eating Let's Do Lunch™ because all the foods taste great and I believe they are healthier and safer than eating all those fattening foods you have thrown away.

Likewise, throw away all the fat-free foods you have in your home that have sugar in them (look on the label under "Ingredients"), except, of course, for sauces and condiments listed in the Grocery Shopping chapter. (Sugar has no fat grams, yet in your body sugar turns to pure fat, and food with sugar in it causes extreme cravings for all the wrong foods!)

Also, after throwing a party, throw away all the fattening foods that have been left over.

The reason for the above is simple – if you don't have any fattening food around, your cravings can't get the best of you. Believe me when I say that if you do keep fattening foods around, eventually you will eat them – especially if you have an occasional drink, which I have found breaks down willpower and creates unbeliev-able cravings for all the wrong foods.

To say the least, I was very happy with myself - until the day I developed an unbelievable craving for pizza. (A craving is an uncontrollable lusting for something you've found extremely pleasurable in the past.)

It was extremely difficult getting through that one day without succumbing to this craving. Had I not been able to stuff myself according to my program, I wouldn't have made it. That night God awakened me again, this time with the thought that what I was really craving was CHEESE. I ended up eating Borden™ fat-free sharp nonfat process cheese product (the least fattening that tastes the best to me) melted on a fat-free large sourdough hard pretzel and WASA® LIGHT RYE ORIGINAL CRISPBREAD (again the least fattening that tastes the best). I don't remember how much I ate, but I do remember eating enough to satisfy my craving.

NOTE: "The least fattening that tastes the best" means other brands might have fewer fat grams, but they didn't taste good to me. And I knew that if I were going to eat anything on a continuing basis, it had to taste great. Therefore, I tried all the brands available to determine the one that I could label as "the least fattening that tastes the best."

If you don't like something I like, then find the least fattening that tastes the best to you and have at it.

I believe that eating bread is like eating a piece of cake, and I loved bread. I would satisfy this by spreading popcorn out into a large flat bowl and using "I Can't Believe It's Not Butter"® spray or "100% extra virgin olive oil cooking spray" (delicious), or melting (in the micro) a few torn strips of fat-free sharp cheese over the top – or I would eat something else with corn, beans or peas in it. On occasion I would have a Snyder's Of Hanover® large, hard, fat-free pretzel with a slice of fat-free sharp cheese melted over the top in the micro. My cravings for bread were eventually totally eliminated.

One of the ways I can tell whether someone really wants to lose weight is to watch how he/she eats a sandwich – open-face on one slice of bread means he/she is trying to lose weight. Anyone eating a sandwich on two slices of bread is destined for DIET FAILURE! (You get the same taste with one slice.)

The absolute best way to eat a sandwich is to have it served on half of a rye, whole wheat or whole grain bun...with the insides removed.

I overcame my craving for sweets by forcing myself to eat fruits whenever I had the urge for pie, cake, ice cream, candy, cookies, etc. This was extremely difficult at first, but you know what eventually happened? I became addicted to fruit, and I now eat it every single day of my life. For example, when I craved the sweet and cold of ice cream, I ate frozen grapes until I was satisfied.

I handled my desire for pizza and sweets, but I couldn't come up with a thing that would salve my life-long craving for red meat. You guessed it – I had another awakening. This time the concept was that I didn't HAVE to find a substitute for red meat. All I had to do was be smarter about eating it. I ate only the leanest red meat available and I ate it for Let's Do Lunch™ until my craving was satisfied. Sometimes this meant scarfing down as much as two pounds of lean ground beef, with each bite being seduced by on-the-side ketchup, relish, tomato and onion.

My love of salty foods presented yet another challenge. And once again, the answer was in my dreams. Popcorn! When I got a salt craving, I thoroughly enjoyed eating a bag of Orville

Redenbacher's® Gourmet® Smart-Pop™ Microwave Popping Corn (again the least fattening that tastes the best). Would you believe I sometimes happily bloated myself with two bags? I sprayed Pam® 100% Extra Virgin Olive Oil Cooking Spray® on it (I would love to see the look on your face when you taste this...you won't believe it!).

In fact, on occasion, for our Let's Do Lunch™ my wife and I go to an early afternoon movie and fill up on popcorn (no butter), even though there is no protein involved. Obviously, this should not be done consistently, as it is vital to eat some protein for Let's Do Lunch™.

Even though I didn't have cravings for pasta or potatoes, Anita did – and she ate something with corn, beans or peas in it, in order to satisfy those cravings.

Almost all the time, I avoided anything fattening by choosing something else on my program that also appealed to me.

Many times I found myself wanting something really substantial, but not knowing what it was. When this happened I'd simply go through my "Grocery Shopping Guide" until something struck my fancy. If nothing appealed to me, I would look for something on my List of Food "To Go" (both in forthcoming chapters).

The next problem was what to do about eating out at restaurants and while "on the road" at fast food places, like McDONALD'S®.

At a restaurant, I ordered the food the way I wanted it – not the way it was presented on the menu, e.g. instead of "pecan crusted fish" I ordered blackened or grilled fish, with tartar sauce on the side.

Also, I remembered to order my non-fattening food in a way that I'd enjoy it, i.e. adding the least fattening thing possible that made the taste likeable (and I still lost weight).

For example, I ordered:

- Blackened, grilled, baked, or broiled fish, with their tartar sauce on the side. Then, I dipped my fork in the tartar sauce and took a bite of fish.

  In order to maximize my weight loss, I asked Anita if she would help me by bringing along my tartar sauce (again, made with Hellmann's® Reduced Fat Cholesterol Free Mayonnaise Dressing and sweet relish) and a Snyder's of Hanover® large Sourdough Hard Pretzel (No Fat *No Cholesterol* No Sugar) just in case I got the urge for a dinner roll.

- Moo goo gai pan (a chicken dish) or chicken chow mein; but not anything "sub gum" because it has nuts in it (and I always say "nuts" to nuts, because the fat goes right to the thighs and the stomach). However, there's nothing wrong with ordering cashew chicken (because it tastes better) and then removing the cashews.

- An "Egg Beaters®" omelet without cheese but with

tomato, onion, green pepper and salsa, and I asked that green beans and corn replace anything else that was normally served with it (at no extra charge).

- I was never afraid to ask for something that wasn't on the menu, e.g. a veggie plate consisting of corn, peas, green beans, lima beans, pinto beans, cole slaw, cooked carrots, etc.

If non-fattening foods were just not tempting, then I'd choose something fattening that I could turn into something not-so-fattening.

For example, I ordered:

- Fried chicken, and then removed the fried skin.

- Eggplant parmigiana or veal parmigiana, and removed the cheese (eating it only with the red sauce).

- A Cobb salad, without croutons and bacon, and with the dressing of my choice (not always diet dressing) on the side. I loved the actual blue cheese that came on it, but I took most of this off, leaving on a little. Then, I dipped my fork in the dressing and took a bite of the salad.

Also in order to maximize my weight loss, I brought my own "reduced calorie" dressing to the restaurant – or, I should say, my wife brought this in her purse (at which time she had to decide which of

HER things she had to leave at home...yeah, right!). The "least fattening that tastes the best" to me are Newman's Own Dressings®. These dressings come in packets. Anita goes to McDonald's® and buys a dozen or so at a time, and then refrigerates them. Each packet contains enough dressing for two salads. (Don't worry if you forget to bring the dressing – just order your choice "on the side".)

- A tuna salad sandwich, but served open-face, on just ONE slice of rye bread.

- An ordinary omelet (without cheese, but with tomato, green pepper, onion and salsa) or scrambled eggs (with salsa on the side). If the eggs looked greasy, I'd discreetly take several clean napkins and blot as much grease off as possible.

- An Italian salad, asking the server not to bring the bread sticks and to leave the cheese and croutons off the salad, replacing them with additional tomatoes, hot peppers and onions.

- A Caesar salad, blackened tuna Caesar salad or a chicken Caesar salad, without cheese or croutons ON TOP.

Following are examples of what I ordered at fast food establishments:

- At Taco Bell®, a Chicken Taco Salad, without avocado, sour cream, guacamole and cheese (all the "gunk" they put right on top), but with a side order of refried beans (if beans are not already part of the taco salad). Then I'd eat everything but the shell. (YES, you can eat the salsa and mild and hot sauces that are available.) And if one taco salad wasn't enough, I'd order two. To this very day I sometimes order two and scarf them down with sensuous pleasure, leaving the shells on the plate.

- A McDonald's® hamburger, threw away the bottom half of the bun and then took clean napkins and blotted as much grease off the meat as possible.

- A McDonald's® salad with a Newman's Own® Dressing (sometimes even for breakfast).

- A McDonald's® McGrilled Chicken™ sandwich, without cheese and with their sauce on the side. I'd throw away the bottom half of the bun and spread on a light layer of the sauce.

- If I was really hungry at breakfast time and at a place where an Egg Beaters® omelet was not available (like a Perkins® or a Cracker Barrel®) I'd order a regular omelet without cheese but with veggies in the middle and tomatoes on the side, and I'd eat salsa on the top. Or, I'd order scrambled eggs, fried in olive oil (if they made a mistake and fried them in butter, I would discreetly dry them off with napkins to get the butter off). At McDonald's® I'd order scrambled eggs (again drying them off) and an Apple Bran Muffin (no butter).

- When I only wanted a little something, I ordered a McDonald's® low fat frozen yogurt cone, put it upside-down in one of their cups and ate everything but the fattening cone itself.

- At KFC®, I ordered white meat chicken and corn-on-the-cob. I took the fried skin off, and then dried the oil off the chicken and the butter off the corn.

- At a salad bar (fast-food chain or grocery store), I loaded up my greens with tomato, green pepper, onion, beets and three-bean salad (all non-fattening), and then I'd choose a diet dressing. (If I had to choose a fattening dressing because I didn't like any of the diet ones, I'd put it on the side and dip my fork in it for each bite.)

  Eating in a less fattening way at restaurants and fastfood establishments started when I was on my "fast track" to weight loss. But now it is a way of life.

- Breakfast, lunch and dinner weren't my only battles. Whenever I went shopping, ran errands, traveled, etc., I almost always got the munchies. To solve this problem, I took along some grapes, raisins or a bag of Orville Redenbacher's® Gourmet® Smart-Pop™ Microwave Popping Corn.

- Anita always put raisins, grapes or sectioned grapefruit in a plastic bag and ate them in the car (on her way to go shopping or run errands) so she wasn't tempted to stop and buy chocolate or candy.

And right before and during her time of the month, both raisins and grapes quelled her craving for sweets like nothing else could. They still do.

- Cocktails, anyone? Although I am not an everyday drinker, I did find myself with the urge to imbibe every once in a while. However, because I believed drinking severely inhibits weight loss, I basically abstained. When I say "basically abstained", let me reiterate that I did slowly lose my last 40 pounds after adding to my diet the social drinking of wines.

I should mention here that I believe drinking grain alcohol will slow down weight loss even more than wine. (I believe grains are fattening, as I'll explain later.)

After I started enjoying wine again – and keep in mind, I'd already lost 190 pounds – I found that on the rare occasions when I drank too much, it brought on the most difficult cravings I'd ever dealt with. I'd come home after drinking wine and have an almost uncontrollable urge for all the foods I knew I should not consume. And, these urges continued through the next day's hangover. I wanted pizza in the worst way. I would bargain with myself that if I filled up on fruit first (even though I DEFINITELY didn't want any) and then waited for 1/2 hour, I could have a pizza. But when the time came to eat it, I was able to control my desire because of the vast amount of natural fruit sugar in my system.

If I was still hungry, I forced myself to eat soup until my stomach looked like a balloon that had just been filled with water. Or I bloated myself with Orville Redenbacher's® Gourmet® Smart-Pop™ Microwave Popping Corn, put in a flat bowl and used olive oil spray, "I Can't Believe It's Not Butter Spray™", or melted a couple slices of fat-free cheese over the top. And occasionally, in order to really satisfy myself, I ate two or three large "No Fat" sourdough hard pretzels (Snyder's of Hangover - sorry, that's Snyder's of Hanover® is the least fattening that tastes the best), with half a slice of Bordon™ Fat-Free Sharp Nonfat Process Cheese Product melted on each in the micro.

Anita believes in being "safe" and therefore she often drinks a glass of water in between each glass of wine – a super idea for us all!

Finally, in order to get you thinking in the right way as to how to be smart in overcoming cravings, let me answer a couple questions that were asked of me recently.

Question: How do I overcome my craving for a Coke® in the morning?

Answer: First of all, you are probably not craving Coke®, you are craving either caffeine or refined sugar. If it's refined sugar, be sure to eat fruits every day - especially the sweetest ones like grapes, pineapple and watermelon. If it's caffeine, try drinking tea or coffee (as little as possible). If this doesn't work, try drinking 3/4 Coke® with 1/4 Diet Coke® for the first week...then 1/2 Coke® with 1/2 Diet Coke® the second week...then 1/4-3/4...then straight Diet Coke® from then on. If nothing works, go for it - but drink as little as possible.

Question: How do I overcome my craving for a sub sandwich every day?

Answer: You are probably craving bread. (Go back earlier in this chapter to see how to beat this craving.) If nothing works, go for it but throw half the bun away (you get the same taste without it) and be sure to have a sandwich that doesn't have processed meats on it. Stick with meats you can lose weight with (skinless chicken, skinless turkey, etc.).

# chapter four

# Losing Weight, "My Way"

In this fascinating process of dropping 230 pounds, I experimented with foods to see what effect they would have on my weight loss. The result was that I found some fattening foods to be non-fattening and some non-fattening foods to be fattening. Also, I found that there were some fattening foods I just couldn't avoid.

Here are some of the secrets that helped make me slender:

1. Desserts are definitely a thing of the past. But don't be dismayed, because by forcing yourself to eat fruits, especially grapes and frozen grapes, you will actually become addicted to them and you will no longer desire desserts or candy.

In order for you to kick your addiction to desserts,

candy and other sweets, it is imperative that you eat fruits every time you have an urge for anything sweet (no matter what time of day it is). You must keep eating fruits until your sweet tooth is salved.

If you must have dessert, try something like strawberries with fructose sprinkled on them or Sugar Free Jell-O® (with or without fruit in it).

And remember, in my opinion, foods don't have to have fat grams in them in order to be fattening. For example, processed and refined sugars and syrups have absolutely no fat grams in them – yet I believe they are totally fattening. (Therefore, fat-free foods that have substantial amounts of processed and refined sugars or syrups in them are indeed fattening.)

2.   For any snack in between meals:

   A. Carrot sticks and veggies are nice, and you can eat all you want (use a little fat-free veggie dip, if necessary).

   B. Orville Redenbacher's® Gourmet® Smart-Pop™ Microwave Popping Corn (have as much as is necessary to salve your craving for a snack. If necessary, use olive oil spray, "I Can't Believe It's Not Butter Spray™," or melt a couple slices of fat-free cheese over the top).

Only if the above two options are not acceptable do you eat any of the following:

C. A couple slices of Wasa® Light Rye Original Crispbread, each with a slice of Borden™ Fat Free Sharp Nonfat Process Cheese Product melted on top.

D. A Snyder's of Hanover® Large Sourdough Hard Pretzel (No Fat*No Cholesterol*No Sugar), again with Borden™ Fat-Free Sharp Nonfat Process Cheese Product melted on.

E. Nonfat frozen yogurt in a cup (no cones).

If you're going out shopping or running errands, put frozen grapes or sectioned grapefruit in a plastic bag and eat in the car on your way, or bring along raisins or a bag of the popcorn mentioned above, just in case you get the munchies. And remember to do the same when traveling.

3. I deem breads, crackers, pasta and potatoes like eating cake. After about a year into my diet I went to the store to find the least fattening bread that tasted the best, and found an Italian bread with 1/2 gram of fat and 60 calories per slice that tasted terrific. I tested my theory by eating four slices of this bread (adding only a light layer of diet jam) as my breakfast each morning, for two weeks, and what happened? My weight loss HALTED. Therefore, obviously, I stopped doing this and tried to refrain from eating ANY bread.

However, this was impossible for me to do. For

example, when I was not that hungry and only wanted a sandwich, how could I have a tuna salad sandwich without having a slice of bread? However, having two slices was not necessary (I got the same taste with one slice as I did with two). Therefore, I'd simply have my sandwich served open-face on one slice of bread, and eat it with a fork.

When I was at home I ate Wasa® Light Rye Original Crispbread (fat-free and like a huge cracker), but as little as possible. When I had tuna salad, chili or tomato soup I sometimes couldn't help myself. And, occasionally, I also ate it when I wanted a snack. Other than that I tried to abstain from breads and crackers. This meant no rolls, buns, bagels, muffins, biscuits, croissants, crackers, bread sticks, flat bread, slices of bread or breaded food at mealtimes, or anytime for that matter.

If you just don't like Wasa® Light Rye Original Crispbread try a Snyder's Of Hanover® Large Sourdough Hard Pretzel (No Fat*No Cholesterol* No Sugar). Then, ONLY if this is still not satisfactory, find something else that fills the bill from the standpoint of "the least fattening that tastes the best", eating as little of it as possible. And, use only "I Can't Believe It's Not Butter™", diet jam or all-fruit jelly if you must have a spread.

In addition, occasionally I had some "yolk-free"

egg noodles (less in fat grams than other noodles) with mixed veggies, and melted a slice or two of Borden™ Fat-Free Sharp Nonfat Process Cheese Product on top. (Other than this, I stayed away from pasta, noodles and rice because I consider them breads.)

I never was a big cereal eater, so this never presented a problem. However, if I were, I would still have stayed away from them as much as possible, because I consider them breads. If you are craving cereal, then eat as little as possible, yet definitely enough to satisfy your craving, and choose "the least fattening that tastes the best", e.g. Kellogg's® Corn Flakes® or Ralston® Corn Chex® (see definition of "corn" below). If you can, eat it with low fat milk and fructose.

I also didn't eat waffles, pancakes, doughnuts and other starchy grain foods – because they are breads.

ULTRA-IMPORTANT: Some people consider beans, peas and corn as foods that are fattening. These foods are starchy protein vegetables and I believe they are nonfattening and can be eaten until full. I ate oodles and they totally eliminated my need for everything mentioned in number 3 of this chapter.

I ate lots of beans in my soups, beans and peas on my salads, peas and corn in my mixed veggies, corn on the cob and lots and lots of popcorn (according to Webster's New World Dictionary of the American Language, College Edition© 1966, the very first definition of "corn" is "a small, hard seed or seed-like FRUIT," and you already know what I think of fruit).

My mother actually uses popcorn in place of bread, doing things like frying eggs 'over easy' in olive oil and eating them with popcorn on top.

Again, I believe that my innovation of eating beans, peas and corn is the reason I no longer have any cravings for breads, pasta, potatoes, cereals, noodles, rice, etc.!

Most overweight people eat a lot of breads, pasta, potatoes, noodles, crackers, cereals, rice, waffles, pancakes, doughnuts, etc. Eating beans, peas and corn should eliminate your cravings for these foods!

It is my belief that fat-free foods made from cereal grasses (grains) are fattening. Think about it...cattle get FAT from eating grains. And, glue is made from flour, and flour from finely ground grain. So when you eat something made with flour or grain, just think of it sticking right to your thighs and stomach.

It is very important that you understand what I just said. It is my belief that rolls, buns, breads, bagels, pasta, potatoes, noodles, crackers, cereals, pretzels, etc. are fattening...even if they are labeled fat-free!

4.  The only cheese I ate was Kraft or Borden™ Fat-Free Sharp Nonfat Process Cheese Product. And I only ate these to satisfy my pizza and cheese cravings, putting them on Wasa® Light Rye Original Crispbread or on fat-free large hard sourdough pretzels, or mixed veggies. Other than this, I abstained from eating cheese.

    It is also my belief that fat-free cheese is fattening.

5.  Oils are full of fat, so I stayed away from them as much as possible, except that I believe the oils in fish and oils made from fruits and vegetables (e.g. olive oil, soy bean oil and corn oil) are nonfattening and can be used in cooking!

    And I constantly lost weight eating vast amounts of 'vegetable oil' salads as main entrees – e.g. Caesar salads made with olive oil or soy bean oil (including grilled chicken and blackened tuna Caesars) and Italian salads (I love the "all you can eat" salad at "The Olive Garden®"); of course, ordering them without cheese and croutons.

6.  Since I found nothing that my mind accepted as a substitution for red meat, I had to have it often. However, I didn't eat it until I got an ACTUAL craving for it. Anita bought the leanest ground beef money could buy and I ate it until satisfied (with ketchup, sweet relish, tomato and onion) as the protein in my LET'S DO LUNCH™.

    That said, in order to cut down on my red meat

consumption, I learned to eat other things I like with it (less fattening or nonfattening things). I put pinto beans and onions with extra lean ground beef and ground turkey breast and ate this delicious mixture with the condiments of my choice, and I mixed ground white meat turkey with extra lean ground beef in my chili. The beef flavor always overwhelms anything else put with it, and therefore I got the same taste as I would if I were eating 100 percent beef (yet what I was putting in my body was much less fattening).

7. French fries, American fries, scalloped, twice baked, mashed, au gratin, hash browns, pan fried, potato salad, potato tots, potato pancakes, potato puffs, potato sticks, candied potatoes, and potato chips are out. In fact, a small bag of potato chips can almost equate to eating ALL DAY on the Let's Do Lunch™ eating program.

For those people who love potatoes, just don't eat them unless you have an ACTUAL craving for them; in that case try a baked potato with salsa or I Can't Believe It's Not Butter Spray™ or olive oil spray, instead of butter, margarine and/or sour cream.

8. When I was serious about losing weight as fast as possible, I abstained from alcoholic drinks of any kind. However, after I had lost approximately 190 pounds, my wife said to me, "Honey, I don't want you any thinner!"

Like the song says, "Here we go again"– God awakened me that very night with the thought that starting to imbibe socially again would slow down my weight loss. The disturbing thing was that the message communicated to me said to only drink wine and not Brandy Manhattans, Vodka Martinis or beer. I didn't like drinking wine, but on those occasions when I decided to imbibe, I forced myself to drink it. After having done this a few times, I found myself desiring wine and not even thinking about booze or beer. (I had to experiment to find wines that didn't give me a headache.)

And I continued to lose weight (although much more slowly) until I had lost an additional 40 pounds - amazing to me even to this day. My wife was so disturbed by this additional weight loss that she insisted I go in for a second physical (and when she found out everything was A.O.K. she was absolutely dumbfounded). When I thought more about it, the inspiration to drink wine fit right in with everything that had transpired previously. What are wines made from? You've got it – grapes. And, grapes are what? You've got it again – fruit.

Remember, for approximately the first year and a half I basically refrained from drinking, and my weight loss during that time was substantially more each month than it was after I started drinking again.

Also, even drinking wine caused me to deal with many more cravings than I had when I was in abstinence.

9.  I didn't drink sugar-loaded soft drinks on my program and I recommend as little diet pop as possible. I didn't lose weight quite as fast when I drank diet pop. (I realize that some people are addicted to diet pop, and to them I say go ahead and drink what you have to, because you will still lose the weight.) Instead, I recommend drinking distilled water, because there are no dissolved solids in it and, therefore, anything that's in the body that can dissolve in this water will do so and will flush right through your system.

    When eating out at a restaurant, I recommend plain old H2O with a slice of lemon in it, bottled water or tea.

10. I avoided dairy products, except for an omelet for breakfast once in a while (made without cheese, and with tomato, green pepper, onion, and salsa). Some people will want a little skim milk or nonfat milk in their coffee, and some people will want a little one-percent or no-fat cottage cheese once in a while. Also, every so often a McDonald's® Lowfat Frozen Yogurt in a cup (not in a cone) is very refreshing. Again, eat as little as possible, because it is my further belief that no-fat cottage cheese is fattening - as is fat-free yogurt.

NOTE: Also consult your physician or registered dietitian regarding your vitamin and mineral supplement requirement. It may be necessary for you to take a calcium supplement, e.g. a couple of Extra  Strength Tums E-X® Tablets each day.

11. Some coffees such as cappuccino are very fattening, but plain old brewed or instant flavored coffee (regular or decaf) is okay.  However, just like with diet pop, I lost weight faster when I drank distilled water, reverse osmosis water, just plain old H2O (with a slice of lemon in it), bottled water or tea. To those people who are addicted to coffee, I say drink as little as possible.  Also, if you must have cream in your coffee, try to use skim milk or no-fat milk.

12. Fast foods can't be eliminated because of the occasional NEED for fast food – due to time con-straints! (Remember to choose the least fattening food on the menu of all the choices that are appealing.)

13. If you just can't stand eating corn on the cob without butter on it, then by all means use a little olive oil spray or I Can't Believe It's Not Butter Spray™ and enjoy! (But, try to stay away from actual butter or margarine.)

14. Acceptable condiments are barbecue sauce, hot sauce, chili sauce, steak sauce, meatless spaghetti sauce, salsa, vinegar, ketchup and sweet relish (all of these are on my Shopping List that comes later).

15. Bananas and avocados may be okay, but I didn't

eat them because I heard (and I don't remember from whom) that they didn't digest as fast as other fruits and I wanted only fast digesting fruit in my body in order to speed up my body's metabolism. In addition, I didn't need bananas for potassium, as my Let's Do Lunch™ program resulted in an excellent potassium level.

16. I used just enough "reduced fat" mayo to hold my tuna salad together, and to make my tartar sauce.

17. Because I never had a "craving" for them, the following foods were eliminated:

Appetizers
Candy
Chocolate
Cocoa
Creams and creamed foods
Deep fried foods
Fats
Fruits canned in heavy syrup or sweetened
Gravies and dips
Guacamole
Jam
Jelly
Marmalade
Molasses
Nuts and Seeds (All nuts and seeds are also extremely fattening)
Processed meats
Scalloped foods

Sour cream
Sugar and sugar products
Syrups
Toppings

I never ate extremely fattening foods like nuts, seeds and potato chips, because a small portion of these foods equated to my being able to eat all day on Let's Do Lunch™.

If you are craving nuts or potato chips you are usually craving something salty, and I've already explained how to deal with a salty craving (see Chapter 3, "Cravings, Eating Out and Other Diet Dilemmas").

If you are craving avocado, try eating the tuna salad I talked about (made with reduced-fat mayo).

18. Once you have been on Let's Do Lunch™ for two weeks, you really won't be tempted to eat fattening foods – except on those occasions when you have imbibed too much and your mind isn't working properly. If you do get sidetracked, the Let's Do Lunch™ program is very easy to get back on. But please don't use this statement as an excuse to be bad!

19. Six to eight glasses of water per day are not necessary because of all the juices in the fruit that is eaten. However, it is certainly a good idea to drink as much water as you like.

20. My 'fruit and soup flush' is a <u>must</u> the day after you have been bad, in order to get rid of the fattening food you ate the day before and get you back on track and make you feel good about yourself again. Eat nothing but acceptable fruits (including popcorn) and soups (e.g. tomato soup mixed with vegetarian vegetable soup, throwing out the potatoes and the pasta) FOR ONE FULL DAY – <u>as often</u> <u>and</u> <u>as</u> <u>much</u> <u>as</u> <u>you</u> <u>want</u>. Be careful to stay away from soups that contain cheese, oils, red meat, potatoes, beer, creams, milk, butter, margarine, gravies, processed meats and other high fats. (See my Grocery Shopping Guide for acceptable soups and fruits.)

21. Again, try to eat only fruit for dinner.

22. Eat fresh, frozen and canned fruits instead of eating applesauce and drinking fruit juices, if possible. Fresh, frozen and canned fruits will fill you up faster and, therefore, you'll consume fewer calories.

23. Another benefit of eating fruit is that many people with constipation problems (which a lot of older people have) will find themselves becoming regular.

In fact, you may find yourself hurrying to the restroom at first. However, the body should soon adjust to your new eating habits and regularity should return.

24. Anita discovered a fruit & veggie wash at the

grocery store, which she uses to remove pesticides, sulfates, herbicides, fungicides and waxes.

25. When you're not really hungry but you just want to chew on something, put a couple pieces of diet chewing gum in your mouth and have at it.

26. Don't eat between meals unless you are extremely hungry. I play golf three times a week with a large group of friends, and inevitably at the 19th hole many of the guys chow down on burgers and fries. If I'm not extremely hungry, I simply sit and visit while sipping a glass of tea. If I can't stand to wait, I eat a little something with them, e.g. a bowl of acceptable soup.

27. When I was dieting and weighing every day, there were some days I would wake up eight pounds heavier than the day before. To say the least, this was very discouraging. So I just decided not to jump on the scale every day. Weighing once a month is perfect (if you just can't stand it, every two weeks is okay). But please don't put yourself through the misery of weighing any more often than once every two weeks, and don't worry about it when your weight plateaus for as long as two to three weeks - KEEP AT IT AND THE WEIGHT WILL COME OFF!

28. Everyone who has lost "major" weight and gained it back knows the punishment NORMALLY involved in dieting:

A. You can't have enough quantity of foods you love.

B. You have to eat foods you don't like.

C. You can't satisfy cravings.

D. And you can't eat whenever you are hungry.

Every time I think about these things I'm reminded of the security guard gal on "Night Court," sitting at the cafeteria table with a stalk of celery, a couple of carrot sticks and making wisecracks about dieting (funny as ____, but not funny if you're grossly overweight and hurting like _____). Punishing your brain in this way is like climbing Mt. Everest wearing sneakers – you're going to slip and fall (and then the hurt comes from gaining more weight back than you lost).

In order for a diet to actually work for the rest of your life:

A. You must be able to eat until you are full, only foods you love and whenever you are hungry.

B. You don't have to eat foods you don't like.

C. You have to be able to satisfy your cravings.

The Let's Do Lunch™ Program fulfills all of these necessities.

Eating only foods you love is extremely important,

because if you don't your brain eventually will not willingly receive what you are eating and you will go back to your old fattening ways.

Likewise, if you don't eat until you are satisfied, your brain will know you are still hungry and sooner or later you'll go back to those old ways.

Satisfying cravings is also crucial, again because YOU JUST CAN'T FOOL THAT OLD BRAIN!

## chapter five

# Overcoming Pitfalls

Even though the Let's Do Lunch™ program addresses all the MAJOR obstacles involved with losing weight, there are other pitfalls to watch out for:

- If you don't eat fruit every day, you could develop terrible "sweet cravings" that could force you off your program.

  After forcing yourself to eat fruits over a short period of time, you will find yourself absolutely not enticed by things like family-sized chocolate bars, cookies, cakes, éclairs and all the other foods made with processed and refined sugar. When I was 425 pounds, if you put a chocolate bar anywhere within 100 yards of me it would be gone before the wrapper had a chance to settle on the table.

- If you eat large quantities of foods (fat-free or not)

with substantial amounts of processed and refined sugars or syrups in them, it could result in a number of consequences:

It could slow or STOP your weight loss, because processed sugars and syrups (again, in my opinion) are very fattening, even though they contain no fat grams.

It could make you more hungry, with the desire to eat only fattening foods.

It could make you want to eat continuously.

It could give you irresistible urges (cravings) for more fattening foods that have processed sugars and syrups in them.

It could make you easily irritable.

And it could make you tired.

- Drinking buddies often aren't sympathetic to your losing weight, and they make sure to offer you the same kind of fattening drinks you used to pour down your throat. (In my case, someone was always buying me a Brandy Manhattan without my asking for it.)

  If you have decided that in Let's Do Lunch™ you are NOT going to drink, then simply pull the bartender or waitress aside and privately tell him/her that you are going to be ordering screwdrivers (or

Bloody Marys) – but that you want plain orange juice (or tomato juice) delivered instead.

If, on the other hand, you have decided that in Let's Do Lunch™ you ARE going to drink (thus losing weight more slowly), then simply tell your buddies that you have become a wine drinker and order a glass of wine – and give your Brandy Manhattan to one of them.

Remember that drinking will bring on extreme cravings, and will sabotage your willpower.

• When staying at a friend's/relative's home, stop at a local grocery store on the way and buy fruits. Tell your hosts you always eat some fruit, and then eat according to Let's Do Lunch™, remembering how to eat on days when you are going to have to eat protein with your dinner (refer back to Let's Do Lunch™).

# chapter six

# Grocery Shopping

Previously I said I would provide the Grocery Shopping Guide my wife reluctantly uses to buy groceries. (When I say "reluctantly," I mean that if she had her way, there would be no grocery stores – just restaurants and caterers.) Here goes:

When buying hamburger, also purchase ground white meat turkey and ground white meat chicken, in order to cut down on fat as much as possible.

1. Buy sirloin steaks and ask the butcher to cut off the fat and put them through the grinder.

2. Buy boneless, skinless turkey breasts and also put them through the grinder.

3. Buy boneless, skinless chicken breasts and likewise put them through the grinder.

Please Note: The names of foods, menus and restaurants identified in this program were specially selected by me. I found them to be the tastiest and healthiest foods for inclusion in my Let's Do Lunch™ program. None of the brands, menus or restaurants have been paid a promotional consideration to be included in the program, nor does their inclusion in the program constitute an endorsement, recommendation or other suggestion by them as to any aspect of Let's Do Lunch™. *All such products and company names are trademarks or registered trademarks of their respective holders.*

IMPORTANT: PLEASE MAKE SURE YOU ARE NOT ALLERGIC TO ANY OF THE FOODS LISTED IN LET'S DO LUNCH™.

## FRESH VEGETABLES

Alfalfa Sprouts

Asparagus

Beets

Broccoli

Brussels Sprouts

Cabbage, green

Cabbage, purple

Carrots, regular and baby

Cauliflower

Celery

Cilantro

Cole Slaw (pre-shredded, no dressing)

Corn-on-the-Cob

Cucumber

Garlic, whole bulb

Ginger Root

Green Beans

Green Onions

Green Peppers

Jalapeno Chili Peppers

Jicama

Lemons

Lettuce, Iceberg, Leaf, Romaine

Lettuce, Mixed, in bag or loose (Spring Mix)

Mushrooms

Onions

Parsley

Radishes

Red Onions

Red Peppers

Scallions

Shallots

Sweet Onions (none French Fried)

Snow Peas

Spinach

Spaghetti Squash

Summer Squash

Sun-Dried Tomatoes (No Oil)

Three Bean Salad, preferably made without oil (if made with oil, then simply drain the oil off as much as possible)

Tomatoes, Cherry and Regular

Turnips

Watercress

Zucchini

Note: No potato chips, candied potatoes, hash browns, au gratin potatoes, French fries, mashed potatoes, scalloped potatoes, potato salad, potato tots, potato pancakes, and potato puffs. I didn't eat baked potatoes, but if you just have to have one, eat it with salsa, olive oil spray, I Can't Believe It's Not Butter Spray™ or Butter Buds®.

## FRESH FRUITS

Apples

Berries:  Blackberries, Blueberries, Raspberries and Strawberries

Cantaloupe

Cherries

Grapes  (put some seedless in freezer)

Grapefruit

Honeydew

Kiwi

Lemons

Limes

Mango

Oranges

Orange Juice (fresh squeezed is best)

Papaya

Peaches

Pears

Pineapple

Plums

Raisins

Tangelos

Tangerines

Watermelon

## CANNED AND BOTTLED JUICES

Campbell's® Tomato Juice

Dole® Apple Juice

Dole® Pineapple Juice

V-8® Picante Vegetable Juice

V-8® 100% Vegetable Juice

## CANNED FRUITS

Del Monte® Chunky Mixed Fruit, in its own juice

Del Monte® Snack Size Lite Fruit Cocktail, drained

Del Monte® No Sugar Added Canned Fruits (packed only in fruit juices and drained before eating)

Dole® Crushed Pineapple

Dole® Pineapple Chunks, in its own juice

Geisha® Mandarin Oranges (drain and rinse before use)

Libby's® Canned Pumpkin

Lindsay® Olives

Lindsay® Pitted Olives

Mott's® Natural Applesauce

Ocean Spray® Whole Berry Cranberry Sauce

## CANNED GOODS

Bumble Bee® Fancy Albacore Tuna, packed in water

Bush's® Best Chili Hot Beans

Bush's® Deluxe Fat-Free Vegetarian Baked Beans – no baked beans with brown sugar and molasses, or with pork and tomato sauce, or canned homestyle

Bush's® Great Northern Beans

Bush's® Kidney Beans

Bush's® Large Butter Beans

Bush's® Navy Beans

Bush's® Pinto Beans

Bush's® Sauerkraut

Campbell's® Beef Broth

Campbell's® Chicken Broth

Campbell's® Home Cookin Chicken Vegetable Soup

Campbell's® Tomato Soup – delicious when made with skim milk

Campbell's® Home Cookin Vegetable Soup

Campbell's® Vegetarian Vegetable Soup

Del Monte® Chunky Tomatoes, Salsa Style

Del Monte® Cut Wax Beans

Del Monte® Lima Beans

Del Monte® Stewed Tomatoes, original recipe

Del Monte® Stewed Tomatoes, Italian recipe

Garlic, minced in jar (produce section)

Green Giant® Corn

Green Giant® Green Beans

Green Giant® Mushrooms

Green Giant® Peas

Greenwood® Whole Pickled Beets (All Natural)

Healthy Choice® Meatless Spaghetti Sauce

Hunt's® Tomato Paste

Hunt's® Tomato Sauce

Hunt's® Tomatoes, Whole

La Choy® Bean Sprouts

La Choy® Water Chestnuts

Old El Paso® Chopped Green Chilies

Old El Paso® Vegetarian or Fat Free Refried Beans

Progresso® Black Beans

Progresso® Healthy Classics Lentil Soup

Salmon

Swanson® Beef Broth (99% Fat Free)

Three Bean-Salad

NOTE: Nothing canned with fat and no combination foods.

## SEASONINGS

Basil (fresh and dried)

Bay Leaf

Beef Boullion Cubes

Blackened Steak Magic

Blackened Redfish Magic

Celery Seed

Chicken Boullion Cubes

Chili Pepper

Chili Powder

Cinnamon

Cumin

Curry Powder

Garlic Powder

Ginger

Italian Seasoning

Lawry's® Seasoned Salt

Lemon Pepper

Mrs. Dash® Seasoning

Mustard (dijon)

Mustard (dry)

Nutmeg

Old El Paso® Taco Seasoning Mix (also chicken seasoning)

Onion (minced)

Onion Powder

Oregano

Paprika

Pepper (black & white)

Peppercorns (black)

Poultry Magic®

Pumpkin Pie Spice

Red Pepper

Sage

Salt

Thyme

Vege-Sal®


**SALAD DRESSINGS, SAUCES, SPRAYS, CONDIMENTS, ETC.**

Anchovy Paste

Barbecue Sauce, Heinz® or Hunt's®

Beano™ Food Enzyme Drops (That's right, a product that keeps you from experiencing those embarrassing moments after eating something yummy that causes gas. You simply put a few drops on your first bite of the dreaded gas-causer and eat to your heart's content, with no more worry of something leaving your body without your wanting it to. It is available at health food stores and some drug stores. From now on you will be able to eat those wonderful gaseous foods that very seldom crossed your lips in the past.)

Butter Buds®

Campbell's® Dried Onion Soup and Recipe Mix

Chili Sauce

Cocktail Sauce

Cornstarch, Argo®

Dill Pickles

Fruit & Veggie Wash (if not in store, from Amway®)

Fructose Fruit Sugar (in place of refined sugar) to use in tea, cooking, etc. – can be purchased at health food store

Hellman's® Reduced Fat "Just 2 Good" Mayonnaise Dressing

Hellmann's® or Best Foods Low Fat Mayonnaise

Hellmann's® or Best Foods Low Fat Tartar Sauce (I like my own better, made with Sweet Relish and Kraft Miracle Whip Free Nonfat Dressing)

Hidden Valley® Ranch Fat-Free Cole Slaw Dressing

Honey

Horseradish

Hot Peppers

Hot Sauce, Tabasco®

I Can't Believe It's Not Butter Spray™

Ketchup, Heinz® or Hunt's®

Kikkoman® Lite Teriyaki Marinade and Sauce

Kraft® Fat-Free Salad Dressings, French, Italian, Ranch (bottles and/or individual packets)

Kraft® Miracle Whip Free Nonfat Dressing

Liquid Smoke®

La Choy® Lite Soy Sauce

Marzetti® Lite Slaw Dressing

Newman's Own® Dressing

Mustard: French's® and Grey Poupon® Dijon

Oils: Canola (Puritan®), Olive, Safflower, Wesson® Vegetable Oil

Pam® Fat-free Olive Oil Cooking Spray

Polaner® All Fruit Spreadable Jams

Polaner® Apricot Puree Spread

Realemon® Lemon Juice from concentrate

Smart Squeeze® Nonfat Margarine spread

Salsa: Tostito's®, Newman's Own®

Spaghetti Sauce, Meatless

Steak Sauce: A-1®

Sweet Relish

Taco Sauce

Vinegar: Apple Cider Vinegar, Balsamic Vinegar, Nakano Seasoned Rice Vinegar, Red Wine Vinegar

Western® Fat Free French Style Dressing

Worcestershire Sauce: Lea and Perrin's®


## VITAMINS

Multi-vitamin that includes vitamin D and iron

Calcium supplement


## BREADS, CEREALS, GRAINS, PASTA AND MISC.

Substitute popcorn, a large hard fat-free pretzel or Wasa® Light Rye Original Crispbread (I ate this fat-free bread with tuna salad, sometimes with chili and tomato soup, and Anita crumbled it up to use in meatloaf, instead of bread crumbs. I didn't eat it with anything else, because I believe that even fat-free pretzels, breads, pasta, potatoes, cereals and other grains are fattening.)

Assorted Dried Beans with Seasoning Packet

Cereals – I didn't eat them, but if you must have cereal eat as little as possible and try Kellogg's® Corn Flakes® or Ralston® Corn Chex® (sweeten with fructose).

Corn meal (yellow)

Orville Redenbacher's® Gourmet Smart-Pop Microwave Popcorn

Popcorn (kernels only)

Split Peas, green or yellow

Snyder's of Hanover® Large Fat-free Sourdough Hard Pretzels

Wasa® Light Rye Crispbread (fat-free)

Wild rice and brown rice (for stuffed green peppers and cabbage rolls)

Wrigley's® Extra Sugarfree Gum

"Yolk-free" egg noodles (ONLY for a pasta or bread craving - and as little as possible)

In general, I stayed away from breads, rolls, croissants, buns, muffins, biscuits, bagels, pasta, potatoes, noodles, crackers, cereals, rice, waffles, pancakes, doughnuts, etc.

Remember, it is my belief that even "fat-free" breads, rolls, buns, muffins, bagels, pasta, potatoes, noodles, crackers, cereals, etc. are fattening.


## MEAT AND POULTRY

Chicken Breast (without skin)

Cornish Hen (without skin)

Filet Mignon

Flank Steak

Ground Beef (extra lean)

Ground Sirloin (ground after fat taken off)

Ground Turkey Breast (ground without skin)

Lamb (lean)

London Broil Steak

Porterhouse Steak

Roasted Chicken (no skin)

Rump Roast

Sirloin Steak

Sirloin Tip Roast

Soup Bones (with lean beef)

T-Bone Steak

Turkey Breast (no skin)

Veal

NOTE: I stayed away from any meat that was not extra lean or at least lean, i.e. no meat with fat in it, no marbled meat, and no processed meat.


**SEAFOOD** (blackened/grilled/baked/broiled, without added fat)

Atlantic Salmon

Brook Trout

Cod Fish

Flounder

Grouper

Haddock

Halibut

Orange Roughy

Red Snapper

Swordfish

Tilapia

Tuna Steaks or Filets

Walleye Pike

NOTE: No fried or deep fried fish, no fish baked or broiled with fat, no fish in oil, no crab cakes or deviled crab and no scalloped oysters.


## DELI ITEMS

Chicken, Barbecued (take skin off)

Chicken, Roasted (take skin off)

Chicken Breast, sliced, Healthy Choice® (no skin)

Three-Bean Salad (drained before eating)

Turkey Breast, sliced, Healthy Choice (no skin)


## BEVERAGES

Coffee (regular and instant), preferably decaf

Diet Snapple® Iced Tea

Diet Soft Drinks:   Canada Dry® Diet Ginger Ale, Diet Rite® Cola (sodium & caffeine free), Diet 7-up®

Distilled Water

Gallo® Cabernet Sauvignon Wine (for recipe only)

Gallo® Chablis Blanc Wine (for recipe only)

Herbal Teas, Celestial Seasoning®, all types

Diet No-Calorie Green Tea (I heard that this is one of the most healthy drinks you can possibly put into your system).

Mineral Water

Reverse Osmosis Water

Spring Water

Tea, Lipton®, preferably decaf

Tea, Lipton® instant decaf (no sugar)

NOTE:  Remember, distilled or reverse osmosis waters are the best; plain old H2O, bottled or canned water without calories is next best.  Tea is wonderful.  Diet drinks are okay, but I stayed away from all other drinks with calories.


**DAIRY AND EGGS**

Blue Cheese, Crumbled

Borden® Fat-free Cheese Slices

Borden® Fat-free Sharp Cheese

Cottage Cheese, Nonfat – or one percent fat if "nonfat" is not available or you just don't like it

Egg Beaters®

Eggs

Gorgonzola Cheese, crumbled

Kraft® Fat-Free Sharp Cheese

Kraft® nonfat Grated Topping (Parmesan Cheese)

Morningstar Farms® Scramblers egg substitute

Nonfat milk or skim milk (ONLY if milk is a must – and as little as possible)

Nonfat Creamer – Carnation®, Coffee-Mate®

Sour Cream, nonfat

Yogurt, Dannon® Nonfat, plain (again as little as possible, and ONLY if fruits, veggies and popcorn are not acceptable)

NOTE: Stay away from other types of dairy products. Remember my belief that fat-free cheese is fattening, as is no fat cottage cheese and fat-free yogurt.


## FROZEN FRUITS AND VEGETABLES

Big Valley® Blueberries

Big Valley® Red Raspberries

Big Valley® Strawberries

Big Valley® Dark Sweet Cherries

(No sweetened fruits; no fruits canned in syrup; no bottled or canned cherries)

Green Giant® Baby Lima Beans

Green Giant® Baby Sweet Peas – none in butter sauce or cheese sauce, and no creamed peas

Green Giant® Broccoli

Green Giant® Cauliflower

Green Giant® Corn

Green Giant® Green Beans

Green Giant® Green Peas

Green Giant® Mixed Vegetables

(No veggies in butter sauce or cheese sauce; no frozen Chinese-style veggies or Italian-style veggies; no creamed veggies)

Minute Maid® Limeade

Minute Maid® Mango Juice

Minute Maid® Orange Juice


## DESSERTS

Dannon® Light Frozen Yogurt

Edy's® Fat Free Frozen Yogurt

Jell-O® Gelatin, Sugar Free

Sugar Free Popsicle® Ice Pops

Welch's® No-sugar-added Fruit Juice Bars

# chapter seven

# SIMPLE
# Recipes

WHAT DID I EAT?

- Anita kept a huge fruit salad in a large mixing
  bowl in the fridge at all times, so that even in the
  middle of the night I could satisfy my sweet tooth.
  She made it with a fresh cantaloupe, a honeydew,
  two or three apples, one and half pounds of green
  seedless grapes, one and a half pounds of red
  seedless grapes, two or three oranges, one can of
  light mixed fruits (drained) and one can of chunky
  pineapple (also drained).

  She didn't add things like papaya, mangos, kiwi,
  watermelon, pears, peaches or strawberries
  because, after setting, they made the fruit salad
  mushy. She simply added these at the time of
  serving.

- For breakfast I normally ate just fruit, and I ate as much as I felt like. Some days I ate a lot and others not so much. But I almost always tried to eat just a little, in order to get enough natural sugar in my system to eliminate later morning cravings and to speed up my metabolism. For some reason I don't understand, I often felt like eating just cut-up grapefruit. After awhile, I was able to get to lunch without eating anything in the morning.

- Baked apples (or apple slices) with cinnamon and fructose pre-mixed and sprinkled on – when it was time to eat fruit and I wanted something different.

- Sugar-Free JELL-O® loaded with fruit.

- A three-egg omelet without cheese and with tomato, green pepper and onion, and eaten with salsa.

- A mixture of tomato soup with vegetarian vegetable soup, taking out the potatoes and the pasta.

- White meat chicken breast (or turkey breast) prepared to taste like beef. Rinse and pat dry with a paper towel. Sprinkle lightly with Poultry Magic® seasoning on both sides. Brown both sides in a pan sprayed with Pam® Fat-Free Olive Oil. Add a can of Swanson® Lower Sodium Beef Broth (100% fat free). Simmer both sides until tender. Shred the chicken or turkey. Again sprinkle lightly with Poultry Magic® seasoning and simmer 30 minutes more (adding more broth if needed). YOU WON'T BELIEVE HOW GOOD THIS TASTES! I ate it with a mixture of fat-free French dressing and my favorite mustard.

- Bush's Deluxe® Vegetarian Baked Beans were just what the doctor ordered and have a scintillating taste that is just plain addictive (and they are fat-free) – but drain off as much of the sugar-laden sauce as possible. Add corn-on-the-cob and you have one of my favorite meals.

- Do your favorite baked bean recipe using fructose instead of brown sugar and, of course, taking out the bacon and anything else that's fattening.

- Blackened, grilled, baked, or broiled fish. I dipped my fork in on-the-side tartar sauce (made with Hellmann's® Reduced Fat Cholesterol Free Mayonnaise Dressing and sweet relish).

- To make tarter sauce: sweet relish and Kraft Miracle Whip Free Nonfat Dressing.

- Tomato Soup, with popcorn dropped on top or with a large hard fat-free pretzel crumbled and dropped in (both ways are delicious and filling).

- To satisfy a red meat craving, Anita prepared a gigantic kettle of veggie soup (made with soup bones from red meat). She let it set in the refrigerator overnight, and the next afternoon she got out of bed (ha ha) to take off the grease that had collected on top. No actual red meat was consumed and yet it often satisfied that craving. (The only problem I had was having to eat it for every meal until it was gone – so that she didn't have to cook again for awhile.)

- Roger Troy burgers are my favorite home hamburgers, and the recipe follows: Mix 1/2 pound ground turkey breast; 1/2 pound extra-lean ground beef; 1/2 cup chopped onion; 2 tablespoons barbecue sauce; 1/4 cup crumbled Wasa® Light Rye Original Crispbread, one egg white and one tablespoon mustard. Grill approximately three minutes on each side. I ate these without buns and with ketchup, sweet relish, tomato and onion.

- Coleslaw can be bought already "washed and ready" in the produce department. Add chopped sweet onion and half a can each of drained pinto beans, kidney beans and navy beans. Mix with Marzetti® Light Slaw Dressing (or make your own with Hellmann's® Reduced Fat Cholesterol Free Mayonnaise Dressing). Season with celery seed and your favorite seasoning. I fell in love with this delightfully delicious mixture.

- A salad with lots of corn, peas, green pepper, pickled beets, onion, tomato, three-bean salad, and with a Newman's Own Dressing on top or WESTERN® FAT FREE DRESSING.

- The same salad as above, except I replaced the three-bean salad with a little blue cheese or Danita's Salsa (recipe comes later).

- Grilled All-Vegetable Harvest Burgers™ and microwaved corn-on-the-cob. I ate the burgers without buns and with ketchup, sweet relish, tomato and onion, and the corn with Molly McButter® or olive oil spray.

NOTE: If you are going to eat anything really fattening like pizza that you are actually craving, it's an absolute must to fill up on fruit first, no matter how many calories are involved, wait the 30 minutes it takes for your stomach to tell your brain just how full it is and then eat your food. (By doing this, you won't eat nearly as much of the fattening food you are craving and you will feel much better about yourself.)

Following are examples of what I ate when I wanted just a little something for a meal:

- Tuna salad, made with just enough Hellmann's® Reduced Fat Cholesterol Free Mayonnaise Dressing to hold it together and frozen peas (thawed out and blotted dry). I added tomato, sweet relish and onion, and enjoyed it all with WASA® LIGHT RYE ORIGINAL CRISPBREAD.

- Tuna, peas and a couple diced hard boiled eggs, with just enough no-fat mayo to hold it together – salt and pepper to taste and serve with tomato slices on lettuce leaves.  (Great for work.)

- Sliced baked turkey (or chicken) with Borden™ Fat-Free Sharp Nonfat Process Cheese Product melted on, and put on Wasa® Light Rye Original Crispbread.

- No-fat refried beans, heated and put with sliced tomato and onion on Wasa® Light Rye Original Crispbread.

- Borden™ Fat-Free Sharp Nonfat Process Cheese Product melted on Wasa® Light Rye Original Crispbread, with sliced tomato on top.

NOTE: When you come up with recipes of your own, please do me the favor of sending your favorites to me, so I can share them with the world. (Please name each one after yourself or a loved one.) Any recipes you send to me cannot be returned and you won't be compensated for them.

I thank you in advance for doing this for me -- Roger Troy Wilson.

# Let's Do Lunch™ Recipe Index

The next several pages are for Let's Do Lunch™ recipes that you will want to use over and over again.

# BRANDO'S LASAGNA

1/4 lb. ground sirloin or lean beef
3/4 lb. white meat skinless ground turkey (turkey will take on flavor of beef)
1/2 cup chopped onion

Cook the turkey, beef and onion until tender.

1-6 oz. can of tomato paste (Hunt's®)
2-5.5 oz. cans of picante tomato juice (V8®)
1-10 3/4 oz. can of condensed tomato soup (Campbell's®)

Add the above ingredients to the onion, beef and turkey mixture.

12 oz. low fat cottage cheese (1% or lower)
2 T parmesan cheese (Kraft® Fat Free)
1/2 cup egg substitute (Morningstar Farms® Scramblers)
2 T fresh parsley—cut up finely
2 T fresh basil—cut up finely
1/2 tsp. white pepper

Combine the above ingredients and mix lightly. Set aside.

12 oz. fat free or skim, grated mozzarella cheese (Alpine Lace®) 5 medium zucchini—sliced thinly

Place the sliced zucchini in one layer in a 13 x 9 x 2 pan that has been sprayed with Pam® Olive Oil Spray. Follow with half of the cottage cheese mixture, half the mozzarella cheese and half of the tomato meat sauce. Continue with another layer beginning with sliced zucchini and ending with the meat sauce.

Bake at 350º for 40-45 minutes.

# CURT'S SLOPPY JOES

2 tsp. olive oil
1/4 cup extra lean ground beef
3/4 cup skinless ground turkey (turkey will take flavor of beef)
1 cup finely chopped onion
1/3 cup finely chopped carrots
1/3 cup finely chopped celery
1/3 cup finely chopped green bell pepper
1/2 tsp. dried oregano
1/2 tsp. dried thyme
1-14 1/2 oz. can whole tomatoes-Hunt's® Blended
2 T tomato paste-Hunt's®
1 T Worcestershire sauce
1/4 tsp. hot sauce
2 baked Idaho potatoes

In medium sauce pan or frying pan heat Oil; add onions, celery, carrots and bell pepper; saute until onions are translucent (about 10 minutes); add oregano, thyme, beef and turkey; saute until beef and turkey are done; add tomatoes, tomato paste, Worcestershire and hot sauce; bring to boil; lower heat and simmer approximately 15 to 20 minutes stirring occasionally; salt and pepper to taste; serve on small baked potato.

Can be served as a lettuce wrap, or to satisfy a bread craving serve in half of a whole wheat, rye or whole grain bun with the insides removed.

# DAD'S STUFFED PEPPERS

6 medium green peppers
1/2 lb. extra lean ground beef
1/2 lb. white meat skinless ground turkey
        (turkey will take on the flavor of beef)
1/3 cup chopped onions
2 cups stewed tomatoes
  (Del Monte Original Recipe)
3/4 cup packaged Success
      or Uncle Ben's brown rice
2 T worcestershire sauce
1 cup fat free grated cheddar
      cheese (Alpine Lace® Cheese)
Salt and pepper

Cut off tops of green pepper and clean and precook in boiling water 5 minutes. Drain.

Brown beef, turkey and onions in a no-stick pan or one sprayed with nonfat vegetable spray. Add tomatoes, rice, worcestershire sauce and salt and pepper to taste. Cover and simmer until rice is almost tender (about 10 minutes). Add grated cheese. Stuff peppers. Stand upright in 10 x 6 x 1 1/2 inch baking dish. Bake uncovered 350º for 45 minutes.

Can be eaten with ketchup.

Great Leftovers.

# DAYNE'S MAIN DISH MEXICAN CHILI

3/4 lb. white meat skinless ground turkey
      (turkey will take on the flavor of beef)
1/4 lb. ground sirloin or lean beef
1/2 cup chopped onion
2-14 oz. cans stewed tomatoes (Del Monte®)
1-15 oz. can kidney beans (Bush's®)
1 cup salsa (Tostitos® or Newman's Own®)
1 cup chopped celery
1 chopped green pepper
1 tsp. chili pepper
1/2 tsp. salt
1/2 tsp. pepper

Cook turkey and beef with onions until browned
thoroughly in a large pan. Add the remaining ingredients.
Simmer.

# DRAY'S BARBECUE

3/4 lb. white meat skinless ground turkey (turkey takes on flavor of beef)
1/4 lb. ground sirloin or lean ground beef
1 cup pineapple juice (Dole ®100% unsweetened)
1/2 cup chopped fresh green peppers
1/2 cup chopped onions
1 T dijon mustard
1 T Worcestershire sauce
1 1/2 cup picante tomato juice (V8®)
1 T cornstarch
1/4 cup water

Cook the turkey and beef until browned. Add onions, green peppers and saute together with the meat. Once tender add the pineapple juice, mustard, Worcestershire sauce and tomato juice. Mix the corn starch in the water. Add to the turkey mixture and  cook to thicken. Serve hot over <u>small</u> amount of Success® or Uncle Ben's® Brown Rice.

Can be served as a lettuce wrap or to satisfy a bread craving serve in a half of a whole wheat, rye or whole grain bun with the insides removed.

## JERRY'S EASY BEEF STEW

2 lbs. very lean beef stew meat
1-28 oz. can tomatoes with juice (Hunt's®)
2 sliced medium onions
2 cups fresh sliced carrots
2 cups fresh sliced celery
1-6 oz. jar sliced mushrooms (Green Giant®)
1-14.5 oz. can green beans (Green Giant®)
1 lb. package frozen peas (Green Giant®)
3 T all-purpose flour
1 tsp. thyme
1 bay leaf
1 T salt
2 minced garlic cloves
1-1.15 oz. package dry onion soup mix (Campbell's®)

Heat dutch oven to 325.º Cut stew meat in 1 inch cubes.
Place meat, tomatoes, onions, carrots, celery, mushrooms
and beans in dutch oven.

Add the following to stew: Flour, thyme, salt, garlic, onion
soup mix and bay leaf.

Cover and bake for 4 hours or until meat is tender.
When done add package of frozen peas.

Serve in a bowl like soup, or over small amount of Success®
or Uncle Ben's® Brown Rice.

# NEET'S MEATLOAF

2 eggs
2/3 cup skim milk
1/4 tsp. pepper
2 tsp. salt
1 medium chopped onion
3 slices Wasa® Lite Rye Crispbread crumbled
1/2 cup finely chopped carrots
1 cup chopped fresh portabella mushrooms
1 cup crumbled blue or gorgonzola cheese
1 lb. ground turkey breast (skinless)
1 lb. lean ground sirloin

Beat eggs slightly. Add seasoning, milk, Wasa® crumbs, onions, carrots, mushrooms, cheese, beef and turkey.

Pre-heat oven to 350°. Form into 1 round loaf on pie pan, or 4 individual oblong loaves in 9 x 13 pan.

Bake 1 hour for round loaf, or 45 minutes for oblong loaves.

Sauce to be spread over meatloaf for the last 10 minutes of baking:

1/4 cup fructose
1/4 cup catsup
1 T. prepared mustard

Mix all ingredients together.

# ROGER TROY BURGERS

Mix 1/2 pound skinless turkey breast, 1/2 pound extra-lean ground sirloin, 1/2 cup chopped onion, 2 tablespoons barbecue sauce, 1/4 cup crumbled Wasa® Light Rye Original Crispbread, one egg white and one tablespoon mustard. Grill approximately three minutes on each side. I ate these WITHOUT BUNS and with ketchup, sweet relish, tomato and onion..and sometimes mustard.

# RON'S AWESOME CHILI

3/4 lb. ground turkey (white meat
        skinless)
1/4 lb. lean ground beef or sirloin
1 cup fresh chopped celery
1/2 cup fresh chopped green pepper
1 chopped onion
1-16 oz. kidney beans (Bush's®)
1-15 oz. chili hot beans (Bush's®)

2-28 oz. cans whole tomatoes, cut up
2 T chili powder
1 tsp. salt
1 bay leaf

Brown meat and onions. Add remaining ingredients. Simmer, covered, three hours.

Great leftovers—this dish freezes well.

# R.M.'s MADE RIGHTS
(Try It—You'll Love It!)

2/3 lb. ground sirloin or extra lean ground beef
2 lb. ground turkey (turkey will take on the flavor of the beef)
1 medium onion—chopped finely
1/2 cup solidly packed 100% natural pumpkin
1 10 3/4 oz. can condensed tomato soup—Campbell's®
1 12 oz. jar chili sauce
1 tsp. pumpkin pie spice
1 tsp. pepper
1 tsp. salt

Brown turkey and beef. Add onions and cook until done. Drain off liquids. Add remaining ingredients and simmer for 1 hour.

Great leftovers.

Can be served as a lettuce wrap or to satisfy a bread craving serve in a half of a whole wheat, rye or whole grain bun with the insides removed.

# STEVE O'S CABBAGE ROLLS

1 large head cabbage (washed)
1/2 lb. ground turkey breast (skinless)
1/2 lb. ground lean sirloin
1 egg, beaten
1/4 cup skim milk
1/4 cup onion—chopped finely
1 tsp. salt
1 cup cooked brown rice (Success® or Uncle Ben's®)

Mix all ingredients together, except for cabbage.

Boil or microwave cabbage approx. 10 minutes or until you can easily remove a leaf. Then remove core, to make it easier to remove leaves.

Make cabbage rolls by forming a small handful of mixture and putting in a cabbage leaf and rolling up.

Place cabbage rolls in a slow cooker. Add sauce (see below) on top and cook on low 7 to 9 hours.

Sauce:

1-16oz. tomato sauce
2 T fructose
2 T lemon juice
2 tsp. Worcestershire Sauce

Mix together all sauce ingredients.

# SHARON'S SPAGHETTI WITH OR WITHOUT MEATBALLS

Sauce:

1 cup finely chopped onion
2 cloves garlic, pressed
1- 28 oz. can tomatoes, chopped
1-15 oz. can tomato sauce
1/4 tsp. black pepper
1 tsp. oregano leaves
1 tsp. salt (optional)
1 tsp. basil
1 tsp. herb seasoning
1 tsp. celery flakes
1 T olive oil
1 bay leaf
1/2 tsp. crushed red pepper

In a large saucepan, saute onion and garlic in oil until tender. Add remaining ingredients. Simmer uncovered until sauce has thickened (30 to 50 minutes). Makes 4 cups.

Serve on spaghetti squash:
Place squash in oven in pan or on foil. Prick with fork to allow steam to escape. Bake at 350° until you can easily stick a fork in it. Cut in half and remove seeds. Scrape out spaghetti squash with a fork.

Meatballs:
1/2 lb. lean  ground sirloin
1/2 lb. ground turkey breast (no skin)
1/2 cup Wasa® Lite Rye Crispbread crumbled
1/4 cup skim milk
2 T finely chopped onion
1 tsp. salt
1/2 tsp. Worcestershire sauce
1 egg

Mix ingredients. Shape into twenty 1 1/2 inch meatballs. Cook over medium heat- turning occasionally until brown, about 20 minutes. Cook in pan in oven at 400° until light brown, 20 to 25 minutes.

# TY'S BEEF, BEANS & TURKEY

1/2 lb. lean ground sirloin
1/2 lb. ground turkey breast (skinless)
1 cup chopped onion
2 or 3-16 oz. cans pinto beans (Bush's® Best, drained well)

Brown beef & turkey. add onions and cook until done.
Drain off liquids. Add drained pinto beans & simmer for
approx. half hour. Season to taste. (Can be served with
Danita's Salsa on top, or with your favorite condiments.)

# BB's CHICKEN WITH MARMALADE

(Try It—You'll Love It!)

1/2 cup of Orange All Fruit Marmalade (Polaner®)
1/2 cup of Fat Free Ranch Dressing (Kraft®)
1/2 cup of Mandarin Oranges, drained (Geisha®)
1/2 package of dried onion soup mix (Campbell's®)
4 boneless, skinless, split chicken breasts

Place chicken breasts in a 9 x 9 pan sprayed with Pam®
Olive Oil Cooking Spray. Cook for 20 minutes at 375.º Drain
off liquid. Blend the marmalade, dressing and dried onion
soup mix together in a blender. Pour over the chicken
breasts. Cook at 375º for another 20 to 30 minutes or until
chicken is tender. Add the mandarin oranges during the last
5 minutes of cooking time.

# BOB'S CHICKEN KEY LIME

4 boneless, skinless split chicken breasts
1-6 oz. can frozen lime juice (Minute Maid®)
2 T honey
1/4 cup pineapple juice, unsweetened (Dole®)
1 T Lea & Perrins® Worcestershire sauce
1 tsp. lemon pepper
2 T cornstarch
4 pineapple slices

Place chicken in a shallow baking dish or pan which has
been sprayed with a no-stick spray. Bake at 375° for 20
minutes, then drain off liquid. Blend the remaining
ingredients (except pineapple slices) in a blender and pour
over the chicken. Bake at 375° for 25 minutes or until
chicken is done. In the last 5 minutes of cooking time, add
pineapple slices to chicken.

## EDNA RUTH'S CHICKEN OR TURKEY... MADE TO TASTE LIKE BEEF

Skinless, boneless chicken breast (or turkey breast). Rinse and pat dry with a paper towel. Sprinkle lightly with Poultry Magic® seasoning on both sides. Brown both sides in a pan sprinkled with Pam® Olive Oil. Add a can of Swanson® Lower Sodium Beef Broth. Simmer both sides until tender. Shred the chicken or turkey. Again sprinkle lightly with Poultry Magic® seasoning and simmer 30 minutes more (adding more broth if needed). YOU WON'T BELIEVE HOW GOOD THIS TASTES! I ate it with a mixture of fat-free French dressing and my favorite mustard.

# ELI'S CHICKEN BREAST ITALIAN

4 split chicken breasts -  skinless, boneless
1-14 1/2 oz. can stewed tomatoes Italian recipe - Del
Monte®
1-6 oz. jar sliced mushrooms - Green Giant®
Parmesan cheese - Kraft® fat free

Preheat oven to 350°
Wash chicken and pat dry with paper towels. Sprinkle lightly with salt and pepper. Place in 10 x 7 oblong baking dish.
Cover with tomatoes and mushrooms and sprinkle top with
parmesan cheese. Cover with foil and bake one hour or
until chicken is done.

# GAYLE'S CHICKEN WITH CRANBERRIES AND ORANGES

## (A Great Dish For Company!)

Preheat Oven to 350°
4 split boneless, skinless chicken breasts
Lawry's Seasoned Salt

Sauce: (Mix and refrigerate the night before)
1-11 oz. can mandarin oranges—Geisha®, drained
1/2-16 oz. can whole berry cranberry sauce—Ocean
Spray®
4 oz. Fat Free French Style Dressing—Western®
1/2 package-1.15 oz. pkg. dry onion soup—Campbell's®

Place chicken breasts in baking dish with lid. Bake for
30 minutes. Remove from oven. Drain off excess liquid.
Sprinkle chicken on one side with Lawry's® Seasoned Salt.
Place chicken in baking dish, smother in 1/2 of the sauce.
(Freeze remaining sauce so that it may be used later.) Bake,
uncovered, at 350° for approximately 30 minutes until
chicken is thoroughly cooked and sauce is hot.

# JACK'S CHICKEN STIR FRY

4 split boneless, skinless chicken breasts- cut into 1 inch
chunks
1/2 cup white wine (Chablis Blanc-Gallo®)
2 cups fresh snow peas
2 scallions - chopped
1 cup fresh carrots - sliced at an angle
2 cups fresh broccoli florets
1/4 cup soy sauce "Lite" (La Choy®)
2 T shredded fresh ginger
1/4 cup condensed chicken broth
1/2-8 oz. can water chestnuts-sliced
1 cup fresh mushrooms

Saute chicken with the wine. Remove and set aside. Place
remaining ingredients in a wok-like pan and stir fry until
just tender. Add chicken and heat until piping hot.

# MARY'S QUICK APPLE CHICKEN

4 split chicken breasts, boneless and skinless
2 T Butter Buds® (liquid)
1 cup apple juice (Dole®)
1 large onion sliced thinly
1 clove garlic minced
1/2 tsp. thyme
4 tsp. dijon mustard
1 large apple, cored and thinly sliced

Flatten chicken breasts in a large non-stick skillet. Add
Butter Buds®. Brown chicken. Add apple juice, onions,
garlic and thyme. Cover 10 to 12 minutes. Remove chicken,
keep warm. Bring liquid to a boil. Add mustard and apple
slices, stirring until liquid is almost gone. Pour over each
chicken breast.

# MOM'S CHICKEN CHOW MEIN

4 split, boneless, skinless chicken breasts—cooked &
cut up
1-10 1/2 oz. can condensed chicken broth (Campbell's®)
2 cups water
1 chicken bouillon cube
2 cups onions—chopped coarsely
3 cups fresh celery—chopped coarsely
1-14 oz. can bean sprouts—drained (La Choy®)
1-5 oz. can sliced water chestnuts—drained (La Choy®)
1 lb. fresh sliced mushrooms - or canned
2 T cornstarch

Saute the chicken in a little chicken broth. Set aside. In
large pan, put the rest of the broth, water and bouillon
cube. Then add onions, celery and cook for a short while
until celery is done (approx. 10 minutes). Add bean sprouts,
water chestnuts and mushrooms. Let simmer and stir for
approx. 15 minutes. Add sauteed chicken and mix together.
Add light soy sauce for your own taste.

If it needs thickening, mix cornstarch with a little cold
water and add to chow mein.

Serve over a small amount of Success® or Uncle Ben's®
Brown rice.

Great leftovers.

# RUTH'S CHICKEN DIVAN

Saute the following in 1/2 cup condensed chicken broth (Campbell's®). Drain.

6 split boneless, skinless chicken
   breasts cut up
1/2 cup onion
1 pound fresh mushrooms—
   cleaned and sliced

White Sauce
1/2 cup Butter Buds®
3 T flour
1 1/2 cups skim milk

2-1 lb. packages frozen chopped broccoli
(Green Giant®)—thawed and completely drained
1/4 cup mayonnaise (Hellmann's® or
Best Foods® Low Fat)
6 slices fat free sharp cheese (Borden®)

Line the bottom of a 9 x 13 pan, which has been sprayed with no-stick spray, with broccoli, chicken, mushroom and onion mixture, white sauce mixture and mayonnaise layered across the top. Bake at 350º for approximately 30 minutes. After baking is done, put on cheese and melt. Remove breasts from pan with slotted spoon or spatula. Don't eat remaining sauce in pan.

Great leftovers.

# TYRA'S CHICKEN PARMESAN

4 split boneless, skinless chicken breasts
Progresso® Italian Style Bread Crumbs
1-15 oz. can of Hunt's® Tomato Sauce
1/2 cup skim milk
Olive Oil No Stick Cooking Spray
Basil, Oregano, Salt and Pepper
Nonfat Parmesan cheese

Preheat oven to 400°. Dip chicken breast in skim milk. Coat chicken breast in bread crumbs. Place in 10x7 glass pan sprayed with Pam®. Bake for 25 minutes or until tender. Pour tomato sauce on chicken breasts. Season to taste with basil, oregano, salt and pepper. Sprinkle with grated topping and bake for an additional 5 minutes.

# B-BOW'S BRONZE FISH

1 1/2 lb. Snapper fillets or any mild fish such as flounder,
         grouper or orange roughy
2 T lemon juice
1 T celery seed
1 cup low fat mayonnaise—(Hellmann's® or Best Foods®)
1/2 cup Parmesan cheese—Kraft® Non Fat Grated Topping

Preheat oven to 350º

Mix mayonnaise, lemon juice and celery seed in small bowl.
Wash fillets. Blot dry with paper towel. Arrange in shallow
baking dish sprayed with non stick cooking spray. Spread
mayonnaise mixture on each fillet. Bake for 15 to 30
minutes, depending on thickness of fillets, until fish is
almost flaky when tested with fork. Remove fish. Sprinkle
with parmesan cheese. Return to oven for approximately 5
minutes. Broil approximately 2 minutes to brown top.

Whatever is not on top of fish when done baking, leave in
pan and dispose— DO NOT EAT.

# CHARLIE'S BLACKENED FISH

4 favorite fish fillets
1 tsp. chili pepper
1 tsp. lemon pepper
1/4 tsp. curry powder
1 tsp. salt
2 tsp. paprika
2 tsp. black pepper
1 tsp. garlic powder
1 tsp. onion powder
2 tsp. red pepper

Shake all spices together. Add the fish and gently shake until each fillet is generously coated. Broil until the fish is just flaky.

Serve with tartar sauce (see recipe) or Hellmann's® reduced fat tartar sauce.

## DEL'S GRILLED TUNA

4 approx. 8 oz. tuna steaks
1 T olive oil
Garlic powder
Preheat Grill.

Brush tuna steaks with oil. Sprinkle tuna with garlic powder on each side. Grill approximately 3 to 5 minutes - don't overcook (tuna will be firm to touch and opaque). You may also blacken tuna with your favorite blackened seasoning.

# DAVID'S EASY HALIBUT

4-6 oz. halibut fillets
1 T olive oil
2 T lemon juice
1 clove garlic...finely minced
1 T fresh parsley
1 tsp. black pepper

In a large bowl, combine everything but fish. Place fillets
on grill and drizzle sauce over fish. Grill approx. 4 to 6 minutes.

# GORDY'S BAKED FISH

4 favorite fish fillets
1/2 cup sliced green pepper
1/2 chopped green onions
1/2 cup sliced carrots
1 lemon —thinly sliced
1 fresh tomato—chopped
2 T chopped parsley
1/2 cup chopped fresh mushrooms

Oven 350°.

Place fish fillets gently over two layers of aluminum foil. Surround the fillets with the remaining ingredients. Bake for 30 to 40 minutes at 350° or until the fish is tender and flaky.

Serve with tartar sauce.

# JIM'S GLAZED SALMON

4 atlantic salmon steaks, about 3/4 inch thick
2 T water
3 T concentrated orange juice (Minute Maid®)
2 T soy sauce "Lite" (La Choy®)
1 T honey
2 tsp. olive oil

Combine everything except salmon steaks in a small bowl to make dressing. Place salmon on ungreased rack or broiler pan. Brush with dressing. Broil or grill for 5 minutes. With large, wide spatula, turn salmon over carefully. Brush with balance of dressing and broil or grill 3 to 7 minutes or until fish flakes easily with fork.

# KITTEN'S TUNA AND NOODLE DISH

6 oz. yolk free egg noodles (Mueller's®)
1-6 oz. can tuna packed in water (Bumble Bee®)
1/2-16 oz. package frozen peas (Green Giant®)
1/2 cup sliced mushrooms (Green Giant®)
2 slices fat free sharp cheese (Borden®)
1 T low fat mayonnaise (Hellmann's® or Best Foods®)

Prepare noodles and peas per package instructions. Drain.
Drain tuna well and chunk up. Add tuna, cheese and mayonnaise to hot peas and noodles. Mix together (or if too dry,
add small amount of skim milk); heat and serve.

Season with salt and pepper to taste.

## NANCY'S TUNA ROLL

2-6 oz. cans white albacore Tuna packed in water
(Bumblebee®)
1 cup packed frozen peas
3 hard boiled eggs
5 T low fat or fat free mayonnaise (Hellmann's®, Best
Foods® or Kraft® Miracle Whip®)
6 or 8 large lettuce leaves


Drain tuna thoroughly, thaw peas, and chop eggs. Mix
together with mayonnaise. Roll into lettuce leaves to make
individual servings.

# TOM'S RANCH STYLE RED SNAPPER

4 snapper fillets
1/2 cup red French reduced calorie dressing
1/8 cup freshly squeezed orange juice
1/2 tsp. paprika
1/4 tsp. ginger
1/4 tsp. nutmeg
2 T fresh orange rind
freshly ground pepper

Spray a shallow baking dish with non-stick vegetable spray. Line with the fillets that have been carefully washed and patted dry. Combine the dressing, orange juice, paprika, ginger and nutmeg in the blender. Mix for 30seconds. Pour over the fish. Sprinkle with the orange rind and black pepper.

Bake at 350° for approx. 30 minutes or until fish is flaky.

# ANGE'S CRUNCHY WALDORF SALAD

6 apples of choice—cubed
1 cup finely diced fresh celery
1/2 cup raisins (Sun-Maid®)

Blend together:
1/3 cup mayonnaise (Hellmann's® or Best Foods® Low Fat)
2/3 cup low fat cottage cheese (1% fat or lower)
1 T lemon juice
1 tsp. fructose

Carefully blend the dressing with the apple combination.
Chill.

# FRED'S CAESAR SALAD

1 head Romaine Lettuce

Dressing:
5 oz. olive oil
1 oz. Egg Beaters® or Morningstar
        Farms® Scramblers egg substitute
1/2 T minced garlic
1/4 tsp. anchovy paste
1/2 tsp. red wine vinegar
1/2 tsp. lemon juice
1/2 tsp. black pepper
1/4 cup Parmesan cheese—
        Kraft® Fat Free Nonfat
        Grated Topping
1/2 tsp. Dijon mustard

Beat eggs until blended on high speed. Slowly add oils while continuing to mix on high speed. Mix until smooth. Add all other ingredients one at a time until smooth. May be kept refrigerated and covered for 7 to 10 days. Dressing must be blended each time it's used.

# CONNIE'S COBB SALAD

1 medium size head iceberg lettuce thinly shredded
1 large fresh tomato—chopped
1 1/2 cups diced skinless cooked chicken
2 hard boiled eggs—chopped
1 cup Green Giant® frozen peas—thawed
1/2 cup fresh green pepper—chopped
1/2 cup celery—chopped
1 oz. finely crumbled blue cheese

Place lettuce in large salad bowl. Arrange individually each of the ingredients. Serve with your favorite fat free dressing on the side.

# MARTHA'S BROCCOLI CAULIFLOWER SALAD

1 head lettuce
4 cups fresh broccoli florets
4 cups cauliflower florets
1 bunch fresh green onions—cut up
1 can water chestnuts drained—sliced

Dressing:

2 cups Kraft® Miracle Whip Free nonfat Dressing
(or less if desired)
5 tsp fructose
1/3 cup Kraft® Fat Free Parmesan Cheese
1/2 tsp. salt
1/2 tsp. basil leaves

Pour dressing over vegetables and refrigerate overnight.
When ready to serve, pour mixture over desired amount of
cut lettuce.

# DANITA'S THREE BEAN SALAD DELIGHT

1-15 oz. can wax beans-drained (Del Monte®)
1-15 oz. can green beans-drained (Green Giant®)
1-15.5 oz. can kidney beans-drained (Bush's®)
1/2 cup chopped red onion
1/2 cup chopped green pepper
1/2 tsp. white pepper
1/4 tsp. Tabasco® sauce
1 T Worcestershire sauce
1 cup fat free Italian dressing (Kraft®)
1 tsp. fructose

Mix the three beans together with the onion and green pepper. Blend pepper, sauces and Italian dressing together and coat the bean mixture. Chill. Serve.

# DIANE'S CURRIED CHICKEN SALAD

6 oz. cooked skinless and boneless chicken breast
　　　chopped as finely as possible
1/8 medium size onion—chopped as finely as possible
1 stalk of celery—chopped as finely as possible
1/2 tsp. salt
1 T sweet relish
1/4 tsp. curry powder
3 T Miracle Whip® Free nonfat Dressing—Kraft®

Mix all together. Chill. Serve on bed of lettuce.

# JOEL LYNN'S SEVEN LAYER SALAD

Layer a large glass bowl with the following:

1 head shredded lettuce
4 stalks of celery—chopped finely
1 green pepper—chopped finely
1 stalk green onion—chopped finely
1 lb. frozen green peas (Green Giant®) (green peas will thaw overnight in a salad)
1 cup mayonnaise (Hellmann's® or Best Foods® Low Fat)
1 cup fat free sour cream
1 tsp. fructose

Layer as follows:
Lettuce, celery, pepper, onion, and peas


Mix the sour cream and mayonnaise together for the final layer. Sprinkle on the fructose. Place in the refrigerator overnight for flavors to blend. Serve carefully from all layers.

## MABEL'S APPLE TUNA SALAD

1-6 1/8 oz. can tuna packed in water (Bumble Bee®)
1 small apple—finely chopped
3 level T Hellmann's® or Best Foods ®
Low Fat Mayonnaise

Once the sauce is thickened add the following
(To make it less spicy, cut down on these):
1 tsp. paprika
1 tsp. freshly ground pepper
1/2 tsp. curry powder

Drain tuna and squeeze out all water. Separate tuna by
rolling between hands. Add chopped apple and mayonnaise
and mix together.

Serve on bed of lettuce. Add sliced tomatoes.

# NEET'S WILD RICE CHICKEN SALAD

1 cup wild rice (uncooked...washed and drained)
5 1/2 cups chicken broth (used to cook rice in)

1 boneless, skinless chicken breast (cooked, cooled and cut up)

juice of 1/2 lemon
4 green onions, sliced up
1/2 red pepper, cut up
2 oz. snow peas, cut in 1 inch pieces

Toss cooked rice with lemon juice. Add chicken, onions, red pepper and snow peas. Toss with dressing (see below). Cover and refrigerate for 2 to 4 hours.

Dressing Ingredients:
2 large garlic cloves
1 T dijon mustard
1/4 cup rice vinegar
1/4 cup olive oil
1/2 tsp. salt
1/4 tsp. fructose
fresh pepper

Blend dressing ingredients in a blender.

# PAT'S QUICK COLESLAW AND BEANS

1 pkg. (approx. 16 oz.) coleslaw, washed.
1/4 small red onion—sliced
1/2 can (16 oz.) pinto beans—drained (Bush's®)
1/2 can (16 oz.) great northern beans—drained (Bush's®)
1/2 can (15.5 oz.) kidney beans—drained (Bush's®)
1/3 cup Fat Free slaw dressing (Marzetti®  or
    Hidden Valley® Ranch Cole Slaw Dressing-Fat Free)

Mix coleslaw, onion and dressing together. Add drained
beans. Season with celery seeds or your favorite seasoning.

Refrigerate several hours or overnight.

## PATTI'S REFRESHING SALAD

2 small heads bib lettuce (or lettuce of choice)
2 oranges
1 grapefruit
1 cup 1% low fat cottage cheese
1 tsp. fructose

Wash lettuce and drain. In large bowl, tear lettuce into bite-size pieces. Peel oranges and grapefruit. Over lettuce, tear oranges and grapefruit into bite size pieces. Mix well. Drain fruit juices. Process cottage cheese and sweetener in a blender until smooth.

Mix all ingredients together.

# TYRA'S TACO SALAD

1/2 lb. lean ground sirloin
1/2 lb. ground turkey breast (skinless)
1 Old El Paso® Taco seasoning mix
2 cups or more chopped lettuce
2 small tomatoes, chopped
1/2 cup chopped onion (optional)
1 can Old El Paso® Refried Beans

Brown beef & turkey. Add seasoning mix & cook as package suggests. On a large plate, layer heated refried beans, then lettuce, cooked mixture, onions, tomatoes and top with Danita's Salsa. (Also try chicken seasoning)

# BUD'S BLACK BEAN BAKED POTATOES

4 medium baking potatoes—scrub well and prick
with fork
1-15 oz. can black beans (Progresso®)

Bake potatoes at 400º for approximately 1 hour. Scoop out
insides of potatoes and place in bowl. Mash well. Add can
of black beans (reserving 1/4 cup of liquid to use later if
mixture is too dry) and mash again. Add mixture back into
potato shells and bake in oven at 350º for 5 to 7 minutes.
Season to taste with Veg-Sal, chives or your favorite seasoning. Eat the skins.

# JOHN'S EASY BAKED BEANS

1/2 cup chopped onion
4 cups Bush's® Vegetarian Baked Beans
2 T fructose
1 T Worcestershire sauce
1 tsp. prepared mustard

Mix all ingredients together. Bake in a 1 1/2 quart bean pot or casserole, uncovered at 350° about 2 hours.

# BILL'S BEAN CAKES WITH SALSA

2 cans (16 oz. each)  pinto beans, drained and rinsed
1/4 tsp. liquid smoke
1/4 tsp. pepper
1/4 cup chopped cilantro
1/2 tsp. ground cumin
1 1/2 T olive oil
1 medium-sized fresh jalapeno chile pepper, seeded and finely chopped
1/4 cup finely chopped red bell pepper
2 cloves garlic, minced or pressed
1 small onion, finely chopped
1/4 cup yellow cornmeal
Olive oil cooking spray (as needed)
1 cup Danita's Salsa (recipe p. 145)

Put 1/2 tablespoon of oil in a non-stick frying pan over medium heat. Add onion, bell pepper, garlic and chili pepper. Cook, stirring often, until onion is soft but not browned (about 5 minutes). Place beans in a large bowl and smash coarsely (smashed beans should stick together). Stir in onion mixture then add liquid smoke, cilantro, cumin and pepper. Mix well. Refrigerate until cold.

Spread cornmeal on a sheet of wax paper. Divide bean mixture into 8 equal portions, shape each into a cake. Coat cakes with cornmeal.

In pan used to cook onion, heat remaining oil over medium-high heat. Add bean cakes and cook, turning until golden brown on both sides 10 minutes... If necessary, spray pan with olive oil cooking spray to prevent sticking. Serve with Danita's Salsa.

# DANIELLE'S DILLED EGGS

6 hard boiled eggs
2 1/2 T Marzetti® Lite Slaw Dressing
1/2 tsp. dill
1/2 tsp. salt

Cut peeled eggs lengthwise into halves. Slip out the yolks and mix them with mixer (Danielle says using the mixer makes them fluffier). Add seasoning & dressing. Mix until smooth. Refill egg white halves with yolk mixture.

# OR TRY:

# DECCA'S DELICIOUS EGGS

6 hard boiled eggs
1/2 tsp. salt
1/2 tsp. dry mustard
1/2 tsp. paprika
2 1/2 T Hellmann's® reduced fat mayonnaise

Same instructions as above.

## DANITA'S SALSA
(sometimes I ate this salsa instead of a salad)

1-15 oz. can black beans, drained
1-14 1/2 oz. can diced tomatoes, drained
1 cup frozen corn
1/4 cup seasoned rice vinegar
1/4 cup chopped onion
1 4 1/2 oz. can chopped green chilies, drained
2 cloves minced garlic
1/4 cup sliced pitted olives (green or black) drained
1/2 cup chopped jalapenos, drained

Mix the above all together and set 1 hour before eating.

Note: This is great over a can of pinto beans, heated and
       drained.

# JIM AND SAUNIE'S ANTIPASTO

1-15 oz. can drained green beans (Green Giant®)
1-15 oz. can drained peas (Green Giant®)
2 tomatoes, chopped
1/4 cup red onion, thinly sliced
1/4 cup sliced green pepper

Season with 1/2 - 3/4 cup of Nakano® Seasoned Rice Vinegar Fat Free.

Let stand overnight in refrigerator.

# MATTIE LOU'S CURRY DIP
### (Great for fresh vegetables!)
2/3 cup 1% low fat cottage cheese
2/3 cup Hellmann's® or Best Foods® Low Fat
mayonnaise
2 T ketchup
2 T honey
2 T grated onion
1 tsp. salt
7 drops Tabasco® Sauce
1 level tsp. curry powder

Mix all together in blender and refrigerate overnight.

## MIKE'S VEGGIE DIP

3/4 cup 1% fat cottage cheese
3 T Hellmann's® or Best Foods® Low Fat Mayonnaise
2 medium carrots, peeled and grated
3 small dill pickles, finely chopped
1 T caraway seed
1/4 tsp. pepper
1/2 tsp. Salt Free Mrs. Dash® Fine Ground
Herbs & Spices
1 tsp. parsley flakes

In a blender, combine cottage cheese and mayo, process until smooth. In a bowl, mix with remaining ingredients. (Do not process again in blender.) Chill overnight. Serve with raw vegetables, especially broccoli, cauliflower and carrots. Makes 1 1/4 cups.

# TY'S TARTAR SAUCE

1 cup Hellmann's® or Best Foods® Low Fat Mayonnaise
1/4 to 1/2 cup sweet relish
1/2 tsp. grated onion (optional)

Blend together and refrigerate.

Substitution for above recipe can be Hellmann's® Reduced Fat Tartar Sauce.

# DORRIE'S COCKTAIL SAUCE

1 cup ketchup
3 to 5 T prepared horseradish
2 tsp. Worcestershire sauce (Lea & Perrins)
1 T lemon juice

Mix well. Chill thoroughly.

Note: For a sharper sauce, add 1/4 tsp. salt, 1 T. lemon juice and a few drops of Tabasco® Sauce (or more horseradish).

## BETTY'S BROCCOLI AND CAULIFLOWER SAVORY SOUP

6 cups condensed chicken broth (Campbell's®)
1-16 oz. package frozen broccoli (Green Giant®)
1-16 oz. package frozen cauliflower (Green Giant®)
1 onion chopped
1 cloves garlic, minced
1 tsp. salt
1 tsp. white pepper
1 T parsley

Place all ingredients in a large saucepan and simmer gently for several hours. Serve hot.

# BOBBI'S TACO SOUP

1 lb. ground turkey breast
1 onion
1-28 oz. can plain tomatoes
1-16 oz. can chili tomatoes
1-16 oz. can pinto beans (drained and rinsed)
1-16 oz. can chili beans
1-16 oz. can corn (drained)
1 package taco seasoning
1 package dry ranch dressing

Brown together the turkey and the onion (drain). Add the
canned vegies and stir in the package of seasoning and
the package of dry ranch dressing.

# CHINA DOLL'S CHICKEN SOUP

2 or 3 skinless chicken breasts with ribs
3 stalks celery
1 lb. carrots, sliced
1 large chopped onion
1/2 bunch fresh parsley, chopped
4 chicken bouillon cubes

Place all ingredients in pan with water until chicken is
tender. Remove chicken, chop and discard bones. Return
chicken to pot and season with salt and pepper to taste.
Simmer on low heat for 1 hour.

# DUSTMAN'S TURKEY AND RICE SOUP

1 lb. skinless white meat ground turkey
    (turkey will take on flavor of beef broth)
1 medium onion, chopped
1 1/2 tsp. dry oregano
1 tsp. Italian seasoning
1-15 oz. can Bush's® kidney beans, drained
3 large firm ripe tomatoes, chopped
3 large carrots, thinly sliced
1 large (about 8 oz.) potato, peeled and diced
6 cups beef broth (Campbell's®)
1 cup tomato juice (Campbell's®)
1 cup dry red wine (Gallo® Cabernet Sauvignon)
1 T Worcestershire® sauce
1/2 cup uncooked brown rice
            (Success® or Uncle Ben's®)
2 medium size zucchini, coarsely diced (about 2 cups)
1 tsp. liquid hot sauce
Pam® Olive Oil Cooking Spray

Spray a wide 4 to 5 quart pan with cooking spray. Crumble turkey into pan. Add onion, oregano and Italian seasoning. Cook over medium heat, stirring often until turkey is no longer pink and onions are soft but not browned (about 5 minutes). Stir in beans, tomatoes, carrots, potato, broth, tomato juice, wine and Worcestershire. Increase heat to medium-high and bring to a boil. Reduce heat, cover and boil gently for 20 minutes. Add rice and zucchini and cover. Continue to cook until rice is done (approx. 10 minutes). Add hot sauce.

Great leftovers.

# EDDIE'S HEARTY HOMEMADE VEGETABLE SOUP

2 small soup bones with lean meat
2 -1 lb., 12 oz. can tomatoes (Hunt's®)
1 cup fresh carrots, sliced
1 cup fresh celery, sliced
1 medium onion, chopped
1-16 oz. package mixed frozen vegetables
                                    (Green Giant®)
4 cups water
2 beef bouillon cubes
5 peppercorns
1 bay leaf

In large pot, combine soup bones, water, bouillon cubes, spices, tomatoes, carrots, celery and onions. Cover and simmer for several hours until vegetables are tender. Remove bones and meat. Add package of mixed frozen vegetables and simmer until they are tender. Refrigerate overnight and remove any fat that has come to the top. Heat and serve.

Great leftovers—this dish freezes well.

# JIMBRO & LEELU'S MUSHROOM SOUP

2 T olive oil
1 cup carrots, diced
1 cup onions, diced
1 cup leeks, sliced (tender parts only)
1 cup celery, diced
1 T fresh thyme leaves, chopped
3 lbs. fresh mushrooms, sliced
6 cups chicken stock
1 tsp. sea salt
1/2 tsp. black pepper, fresh ground
4 tsp. chives, minced

In a large stockpot, sauté onions, celery & leeks in oil, until onions are clear. Stir in thyme, mushrooms simmer until mushrooms have softened.

Add chicken stock, salt, pepper; cover & simmer for 30 minutes. Puree the mixture in a blender to desired consistency. Serve hot & garnish with chives.

*"If you like mushrooms, especially in soup, this dish will be a hit with the entire group."*

# JIMBRO & LEELU'S TOMATO SOUP

3 T olive oil
2 onions, finely chopped
2 tsp. garlic, minced
3 lb. ripe roma tomatoes, diced
3 sprigs Italian parsley, chopped
4 fresh basil leaves, chopped
1/2 tsp. cayenne pepper
Salt & Pepper to taste

Sauté onions in oil, until onions are clear. Add garlic & sauté 2 more minutes. Stir in tomatoes, cayenne pepper, parsley & basil. Simmer over low heat, stirring occasionally to prevent scorching. Simmer tomatoes until they have given off their juices, about 30 minutes.

Pass the mixture through a blender until desired consistency is reached. Add salt & pepper to taste. For spicier soup, just add more cayenne pepper.

*"Potato, potata, tomato, tomata, what'a you matta, you no like soupa?"*

# JOANIE'S MINESTRONE SOUP

Make a large batch and freeze individual servings for days when you're on the go.

1 medium onion, chopped
1/2 T vegetable oil
1/4 tsp. fresh minced garlic
1 can (14 1/2 oz.) ready-cut tomatoes (Hunt's®)
   (or 2 cups chopped fresh tomatoes, optional)

1 pkg. (16 oz.) frozen mixed vegetables (Italian style    recommended)
2 cups tomato or V-8 ® juice
1 cup reduced sodium chicken or beef broth (Campbell's®)
1 1/2 tsp. fructose
1 tsp. Italian seasoning
1 T basil
1/8 tsp. pepper
1 can (15 oz.) Great Northern® Navy Beans

In a large soup pot, saute onion, olive oil and garlic over medium heat until onion is soft. Add tomatoes, vegetables, tomato juice, broth, fructose and seasonings.  Bring to boil and add drained beans. Reduce heat and cover. Simmer approximately 20 minutes. If soup is too thick, add more tomato juice or water.

# LOERITA'S QUICK BEAN SOUP

1-16 oz. can Bush's® Pinto Beans
1-16 oz. can Bush's® Great Northern Beans
1-14 1/2 oz. can Del Monte® Stewed Tomatoes
1/2 can water
1 medium onion, chopped


Mix together. Heat until hot and then simmer
approximately 30 to 45 minutes.

# SUZIE'S SPICY BLACK BEAN SOUP

1/2 cup chopped onion
1 green pepper.....chopped
1 cup celery.....chopped
4-15 oz. cans black beans (Progresso®)
1 cup chopped carrots
1 cup frozen corn
2 cloves chopped garlic
1 1/2 fresh tomatoes, chopped (or canned & chopped)
4 beef bouillon cubes
1/2 T cumin
1/2 T oregano
1 T olive oil


Sauté onions, peppers, and celery in oil. Add remaining ingredients. Mix & simmer approx. 1 hour or until carrots are done.

# SHIRLEY'S EASY FRUIT SALAD

1 fresh cantaloupe—cut up
1 fresh honeydew—cut up
2 or 3 apples—cut up small
1 lb. green grapes
1 lb. red grapes
3 oranges—cut up
1/4 cup raisins
2-20 oz. cans chunk pineapple in its own juice
(Dole®)
1-16 oz. can chunky mixed fruit in its own juice
(Del Monte®)

Drain canned fruit and add to fresh fruit and raisins.

# LET'S DO LUNCH™ FRUIT SALAD

Apples
Blueberries
Cantaloupe
Cherries
Grapes, Grapes and more Grapes
Grapefruit
Honeydew
Kiwi fruit*
Mango*
Oranges
Papaya*
Peaches*
Pears*
Pineapple
Plums*
Raspberries
Strawberries*
Tangerines
Watermelon*

Combine any, part, or all of your favorite fruit in a salad!!!

*Some fruits are best combined with the salad just before eating in order to keep them fresh and to keep the salad from becoming mushy.

## LARRY'S 3-EGG OMELET

1 whole egg
2 egg whites
1/4 cup fresh chopped green pepper
1/4 cup chopped onions
1/4 cup fresh chopped mushrooms
1/2 cup chopped tomatoes
1 slice Borden® Fat Free cheese (if a must)

Stir eggs with fork until whites and yolk are blended. In an omelet pan sprayed with Pam®, pour in mixture and cook slowly on low heat. As under surface becomes set, lift it slightly with a spatula to let uncooked portion flow underneath and cook. Add onions,   peppers, and mushrooms. When almost done, add tomatoes and fat free cheese. Fold or roll it and serve immediately with salsa.

# chapter eight

# Food "To Go"

Where did I go to bring something home to eat?

- McDonald's® for scrambled eggs (drying them off with napkins to get the butter and oils off) and an Apple Bran Muffin (no butter).

- Perkins® for an "Egg Beaters®" type omelet (or two of them if I was really hungry), made without cheese and with tomato, green pepper and onion. When I got home I ate it with salsa.

- Olive Garden® for their eggplant parmigiana or veal parmigiana, throwing away the cheese.

- The grocery store salad bar for a salad made with sliced tomato, green pepper, onion, peas and pickled beets, and topped with three-bean salad for the dressing.

- McDonald's® for a Chunky Chicken Salad, with Newman's Own dressing.

- Taco Bell® for a Chicken Taco Salad, without avocado, sour cream, guacamole and cheese, and with a side order of refried beans to put on (if beans were not already part of the taco salad). I added their complimentary salsa and hot and mild sauces, and ate everything but the shell.

- The grocery store for barbecue chicken and three-bean salad. I took the skin off the chicken and drained the oil off the salad.

- KFC® for white meat chicken and corn-on-the-cob. I took off the fried skin and blotted all dry.

- McDonald's® for a McGrilled Chicken™ sandwich without cheese and sauce. I brought it home, threw away the bottom half of the bun and added a light layer of Hellmann's® Reduced Fat Cholesterol Free Mayonnaise Dressing.

- My favorite Chinese restaurant for moo goo gai pan, chicken chow mein or just plain chow mein. I threw away the rice and the "crispies." Sometimes I ordered cashew chicken and threw away the cashews.

- McDonald's® for a burger without cheese. I threw away the bottom half of the bun and blotted dry the meat.

- If I wanted a treat, I went to McDonald's® for a lowfat frozen yogurt cone and put it upside down in a cup. I brought it home and ate only the yogurt – not the cone. Once in a while, Anita took a plastic bowl and had them fill it up. She brought it home in a cooler.

Use your imagination in putting together your personalized list of where to go to bring home something acceptable to eat.

## chapter nine

# Lose Weight, "Your Way"

Now you know the Let's Do Lunch™ eating program. But wait a minute. There's still one more thing you need to know - WHY you must do it your way.

First of all, we are all different from the standpoint of our favorite fattening foods. My favorites were pizza and red meat; Anita's were mashed potatoes (with gravy, of course), chocolate bars and pizza. You will have to deal with any actual cravings for your favorites.

You also must be the one who decides whether to lose weight as fast as you can or a little slower (this can be done by not giving up wine and/or not giving up that one certain food – though you only eat it when you are actually craving it, after first filling up on fruit and then waiting the 30 minutes it takes for your stomach to tell your brain just how full it is).

Further, the "least fattening that tastes the best" of any given food might be totally different for you than what it is for me. Start your program by using my suggestions, and if you don't like something then experiment until you find "the least fattening-that tastes the best to you".

Additionally, something you like that's just a little fattening might very well go with something nonfattening, the result being that it will help you Let's Do Lunch™.

Then there's the matter of leaving from work to go to a cocktail party, banquet, business dinner, travel, etc. In the Let's Do Lunch™ program, you must solve the problem of where to get the fruits you need. Here are some suggestions:

1. Carry a cooler to work, filled with the fruits you like and enough ice packs to keep them cold.

2. Put a small refrigerator in your place of business, to hold those fruits you like.

3. Take to work pop-top cans of fruit (remember to buy fruits that are packed in fruit juices, and drain them before eating).

4. Take fruits like grapes, apples and grapefruits to work (ones that can set all day and not spoil).

NOTE: Remember to take enough fruit to work to actually fill up on (in case you have a craving for something really fattening).

Two other items you should put in your workplace are a small microwave, in order to make popcorn, etc. and a small electric two-sided grill to prepare proteins for lunch.

Now let's talk about Let's Do Lunch™ from the aspect of exercising. When I was losing weight, I didn't exercise – I simply participated in activities I liked. I hit golf balls (although I rode in a cart when I played) and I took a dip in the pool once in a while.

My wife played tennis and walked (because she enjoyed walking).

My mother drove to the hotel on Sundays to indulge in their all-you-can-eat and drink champagne brunch (just kidding) – her exercise was walking out to the driveway every morning to pick up the newspaper (not kidding).

In other words, you can Let's Do Lunch™ without exercising, or you can lose it even faster by engaging in some physical activity, like gardening. In any case, make sure that you like whatever kind of activity you become involved with (this is a must, because you won't stay with it unless you like it)!

Please call your doctor to get his/her approval of the activity in which you intend to participate.

To those of you who are out there walking every morning and just can't seem to lose any weight no matter how many miles you log: you are probably sitting down at the dinner table and eating rolls, bread, pasta, crackers, potatoes, fat-free foods that have sugar in them, etc. I see it all the time - people out there working their buns off every morning and then biting into buns at mealtimes, because they think it's okay as long as they don't add butter or margarine. NOT! I firmly believe that what they are eating is like eating cake. Butter or margarine just adds insult to injury. In general, show me a "fatty" and I'll show you someone who eats rolls, bread, crackers, pasta, potatoes, fat-free foods that have sugar in them, etc.

In the 15 years of experimenting with my own body, I tried to lose weight by exercising – to no avail. In fact, just before the Lord blessed me with Let's Do Lunch™ I had been exercising at least 1-1/2 hours every day, and gained over 45 pounds doing it. With Let's Do Lunch™, it took me just 3 months to lose that 45 pounds and get back down to my svelte self.

What to do when you have reached your weight loss goal (in other words, maintenance): the answer is that you do absolutely nothing! In the process of Let's Do Lunch™ your body weight will eventually level off, you will look terrific, and you just continue eating in the same way as you have been – on YOUR program.

If you want to gain a few pounds (FAT CHANCE) because you have lost too much weight, then have fun by adding an occasional fattening food. (How brilliant

I am!)

The biggest problem you are going to have is believing that you can eat every time you are hungry, eat until you are full, eat only foods you love AND STILL LOSE WEIGHT!

You will be talking to yourself, saying things like, "I can't eat all these grapes - there are 100 calories in every 10 to 12 of them. I'm only going to eat just a few." Or, "I can't eat three hamburger patties for lunch - too many calories and fat grams involved. I'm only going to eat one patty."

If this is what you're going to do, then don't bother with Let's Do Lunch™. You are destined for failure. So, even though I say to do it "your way," the one thing you MUST strictly do is adhere to God's KEY that ultimately made all the difference in the world in my losing weight – Let's Do Lunch™.

What a diet! Whenever you are hungry, eating foods you love until you are full. I can hear my critics now - this guy must be spending time in "La La Land"! Again I say, I'm telling the truth. And as I said before, I have many distinguished friends and family (including my doctors) who will attest to witnessing my weight loss. Further, my mother, my wife, my agent and I are living testimonials to the ideas that God gave me in the middle of nights.

I wouldn't believe it either if it hadn't happened to me. But it did, and now IT IS MY DESTINY to devote the rest of my life to helping take away the tears like I have seen on the faces of all the heavy women, children and men who have "told it like it is" on all the TV talk shows.

And then there are those who have held their tears inside. I remember the time I sat at home in the solitude of my bedroom, looked down at my 5-foot stomach and realized that I just couldn't lose weight. I used to joke about it and laugh at jokes about it. I even used to tell people that being fat was okay (it was like being tall or short). But deep inside I was hurting so much that I just wanted to die and go to heaven. And that hurt deepened each time I went out to a restaurant and saw people glaring at me, and heard their whispers.

My life has totally changed since then. But that's another story, and I wanted to keep this book to a minimum (every diet book I have ever seen was so thick and so detailed I just didn't want to pick it up).

YOU ARE NOW READY TO START WHAT WILL BE THE MOST WONDERFUL VENTURE OF YOUR LIFE, and you are going to make heads turn ... and when you do, please remember to say a little prayer ... thanking God for His Diet. (It's not my diet – He's the One who awakened me in the middle of many nights with the ideas that saved my life.)

NOTE: Once you have lost weight, if you have children in school please pick up your phone and call a member of your school board to explain Let's Do Lunch™, and then loan that person this book. Hopefully, this will start a "grass roots" campaign to change our school lunch programs to Let's Do Lunch™ programs.

I hope to see you at one of my personal appearances in the near future - in a slimmer body, of course. In that case, Let's Do Lunch™.

The best of luck, and let me know how you're doing.

Roger Troy Wilson

**Sunshine Publications, Inc.**
**23924 Creek Branch Lane**
**Bonita Springs, FL 34135**

**P.S. Please see next chapter**

# chapter nine

# Diary, Notes, Personal Recipes

Use the following pages to keep track of your progress, to make notes of your own experiences and discoveries. Also, add your personal recipes.

NOTE: Again I ask that when you come up with recipes of your own, please do me the favor of sending your favorites to me, so I can share them with the world. (Please name each one after yourself or a loved one.)

Any recipes you send to me cannot be returned and you won't be compensated for them.

Again I thank you in advance for doing this for me.

Roger Troy Wilson